THE CHILDREN ACT AND MEDICAL PRACTICE

Barbara Mitchels LLB, Solicitor
DIP COUNSELLING AND PSYCHOTHERAPY

Alister Prince B TECH, Social Worker
DIP APP SOC STUDIES, CQSW, MPPS

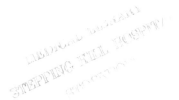

FAMILY LAW
1992

Published by
Jordan & Sons Ltd
21 St Thomas Street
Bristol BS1 6JS

© Jordan & Sons Ltd 1992

British Library Cataloguing-in-Publication Data
A catalogue record for this book is available from the British Library.

ISBN 0 85308 142 5

Typeset by Rowland Phototypesetting Ltd, Bury St Edmunds, Suffolk.
Printed in Great Britain by Henry Ling Limited, The Dorset Press, Dorchester.

FOREWORD

Most of us work best and are more comfortable in familiar surroundings – however unfriendly those surroundings may seem to others. Most doctors feel comfortable in any hospital or health centre, but when displaced into a school, a department of social services or, worst of all, a court of law, will be ill at ease.

Yet all those who work on behalf of children and with families, recognise that it is imperative to liaise closely with people from other disciplines and to be able to work effectively on other people's territory.

Moreover, in the same way that doctors have traditional methods of working, so do lawyers and so do social workers. Each profession adheres to methods that are tried and trusted and often there are difficulties in understanding the ways in which other disciplines function.

This book will help us to understand each other better and to know each other's strengths and limitations. It is written by a lawyer and a social worker, both of whom have extensive experience of inter-disciplinary work and of child care legislation. It is written clearly, and with sympathy, in a way that will make life easier for everyone who is either irritated by the law or feels threatened when participating in court proceedings. The authors explain not only current child care legislation, including the changes resulting from the Children Act 1989, but also the way in which the courts work. As a practitioner's guide it should enable us all to work more effectively for children and their families.

ROY MEADOW
Leeds
October 1992

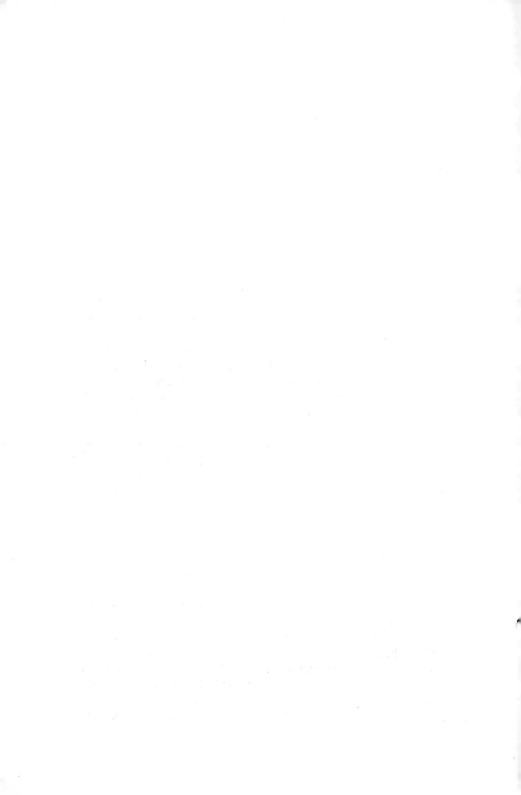

PREFACE

The Children Act 1989 ('the Act') makes radical changes in the law relating to children and their families. In medical and psychiatric practice, these changes necessarily affect many aspects of work, including record-keeping, medical consents for examination and treatment, and also the preparation of reports for court. The changes are not only in the law, but also in our approach to child protection and child care. Openness, co-operation and negotiation are vital. Wherever possible, the legislation encourages children to remain within their own families with the provision of advice and resources to make this possible. Health care is one of these vital resources.

Case-law provides the interpretation of legislation. During the year since the Act came into force, the courts have had to adjudicate in many situations presenting legal, ethical and moral dilemmas, one of which is the extent of control which a court may exercise in medical matters, and the circumstances in which a court can or should overrule a person's expressed wish concerning medical treatment.

In a series of decisions concerning medical consent, the courts have demonstrated their power to protect children by authorising or refusing medical treatment. In one recent case, a blood transfusion was authorised, and in another, the court refused to sanction artificial ventilation requested for a child by relatives because a consultant paediatrician advised that this would not be in the child's best interests.

The courts frequently make medical decisions for mentally incapacitated adults, but in two very recent cases, this has been extended to adults who were not mentally ill within the terms of the Mental Health Acts, but who had refused treatment on religious grounds. Sir Stephen Brown, on 12 October 1992, authorised a caesarian section against the wishes of the patient (who had refused the operation on religious grounds) on the basis that the operation was necessary in an attempt to save the lives of both the mother and her unborn child. This decision, as yet unreported, is, so far as the authors are aware, the first of its kind in English legal history.

Lawyers often struggle with medical terminology. Doctors often find litigation frustrating and incomprehensible. Both professions have difficulty in meeting each other's needs in the preparation of court cases because their respective disciplines are so different. We hope that this book will go some way towards creating an understanding of the new legislation as it affects medical practice, and how doctors and lawyers can help each other in the litigation process.

The Act makes changes in private law where it applies between individuals, and in public law where the State intervenes in the life of a family or an individual. There is frequently an overlap in public and private law in respect of children. The court has to consider all the available options when making decisions about a child. Practitioners need to know about public law and child protection and about the various private law alternatives open to the court.

Legislation usually refers to individuals as 'he' and 'him', and to those under the age of 18 as 'children'. We unreservedly apologise to the large proportion of the population who are not covered by this terminology for having to follow this precedent, and it goes without saying that we wish our text to be read as including everyone to whom it applies.

For the sake of brevity we have used the term 'practitioners' throughout the book to include medical and mental health workers, doctors, dentists, psychiatrists, counsellors, psychotherapists, nursing and paramedical staff, and others involved in the health care of children and their families.

We are both committed to the enhancement of communication between different disciplines and we would welcome feedback from practitioners with guidance, suggestions for further topics, specific requirements and, of course, constructive criticism.

Alister wishes to thank Peter Goodall for all his hard work, and we would both like to acknowledge with gratitude the patience, tolerance and support of our families and friends.

BARBARA MITCHELS AND ALISTER PRINCE
14 October 1992

CONTENTS

FOREWORD   v
PREFACE   vii
CONTENTS   ix

Chapter 1   GENERAL PRINCIPLES UNDERLYING THE
            CHILDREN ACT 1989   1
            Partnership and co-operation   1
            Avoidance of delay   1
            Concurrent powers   2
            The child is a person, not an object of concern   2
            The welfare of the child is the court's paramount
            consideration   3
            Welfare checklist   3
            Non-intervention   4
Chapter 2   PARENTAL RESPONSIBILITY   7
            What is parental responsibility?   7
            Who has parental responsibility?   9
            What does parental responsibility allow one to do? 12
            Parental responsibility and medical records   12
            Parental responsibility agreement   13
Chapter 3   RESIDENCE AND CONTACT ORDERS   15
            Local authority may not use residence or section 8
            contact orders   15
            Limitations for children in statutory care of local
            authority   16
            Residence orders   16
            Contact orders   19
            Contact with children in statutory care   21

Chapter 4   SPECIFIC ISSUE AND PROHIBITED STEPS
             ORDERS   23
             Specific issue orders   24
             Prohibited steps orders   26
Chapter 5   EMERGENCY PROTECTION ORDERS   29
             Introduction   29
             Who may apply?   29
             Significant harm   30
             Timing of the order   30
             Consequences of the order   31
             The role of medical practitioners and psychiatrists   31
             Conclusion   33
Chapter 6   POLICE PROTECTION   35
             Extent of police powers   35
             Time-limits   35
             Who must be informed?   35
             Further action after implementation of police
             protection   36
             Contact with a child in police protection   36
Chapter 7   CARE AND SUPERVISION ORDERS   39
             Only one route into care   39
             Only a local authority or authorised person may
             apply for a care order   39
             New grounds for care and supervision   39
             Effect of care order   41
             Contact with children in statutory care   42
             Effect of supervision order   42
             Medical and psychiatric examination and treatment
             under supervision order   42
             Education supervision orders   43
             Interim care and supervision orders/medical and
             psychiatric assessments   43
             Duration of care and supervision orders   44
Chapter 8   CHILD ASSESSMENT ORDERS   45
             Introduction   45
             When is an application made?   46
             Steps towards application   47
             Recording the process   48
             Who does the assessment?   48
             Role of the guardian ad litem   49

	Directions of the court	49
	The timing of the assessment	50
	Race and culture	51
	Failure to produce the child	51
	Conclusion	51
Chapter 9	PROVISION OF RESOURCES FOR CHILDREN IN NEED	53
	Introduction	53
	Definitions of need	53
	Discretionary and non-discretionary powers and duties	54
	The register of disabled children	54
	Information about services	55
	The child and the family	55
	Accommodation of children by the local authority	56
	The provision of family centres	57
	The provision of day care	57
	The prevention of abuse and neglect	57
	Race and culture	58
	The role of the medical practitioner	59
	Statutory duty to co-operate	60
	Voluntary agencies	60
	Conclusion	61
Chapter 10	CONSENT TO MEDICAL EXAMINATIONS AND ASSESSMENT	63
	Consents for medical examination and treatment generally	63
	Problem situations	71
	Power of the High Court in wardship or its inherent jurisdiction to override decisions of parents, child or others	73
	The new legislation: specific provisions of the Children Act 1989 relating to medical or psychiatric examination and assessment	73
Chapter 11	COMMUNICATING WITH CHILDREN AND ADOLESCENTS	79
	Introduction	79
	Age-appropriate language	79
	The child-centred approach	80
	Communication difficulties	81

The role of the guardian ad litem   82
The *Gillick* judgment   83
Suspicions of sexual abuse   83
Conclusion   84

Chapter 12   INTER-AGENCY CO-OPERATION IN THE
              INVESTIGATION OF CHILD ABUSE   85
              Introduction   85
              Working together   86
              Area child protection committees and procedures   86
              Training in inter-agency co-operation   86
              The initial process of investigations   87
              Partnership and positive progress   88
              Child protection conferences   89
              The practitioner as specialist   91
              The investigation of sexual abuse   92
              Other forms of child abuse   94
              Institutional child abuse   95
              Race, culture, religion, class, disability, gender
              and sexuality   96
              Statutory intervention   97
              Conclusion   97

Chapter 13   PREPARATION OF REPORTS FOR COURT   99
              Notes and records   99
              Preparation   101
              Format of medical reports for court   101
              Content of reports generally   104

Chapter 14   EXPERT EVIDENCE   113
              Be prepared   113
              Where to go on arrival at court   114
              In the witness box   115
              Payment   117
              Inter-disciplinary communication   118

GLOSSARY   119
APPENDICES   131
              1 Confidentiality and disclosure of medical
                information   131
              2 Annotated extracts from the current edition of a
                guide to consent for examination and treatment
                (NHS Management Executive)   135
INDEX   145

Chapter 1

GENERAL PRINCIPLES UNDERLYING THE CHILDREN ACT 1989

PARTNERSHIP AND CO-OPERATION

The Children Act 1989 ('the Act') embodies radical new thinking about the relationship between individuals and their children, and between families and those agencies whose task is to provide resources and assistance for children and their families. The concepts of co-operation, negotiation, and partnership, together with a more efficient and effective legal framework for the protection of children have led to the development of a number of principles which are set out clearly in the Act and make specific requirements of the court.

AVOIDANCE OF DELAY

The Act commences with a clear direction in s 1(1) (see Figure 1.1), that:

'When a court determines any question with respect to –

(a) the upbringing of a child; or
(b) the administration of a child's property or the application of any income arising from it,

the child's welfare shall be the court's paramount consideration.'

The same section (s 1(2)) also embodies the principle that children should not be subjected to the potential abuse of unnecessary delay in the resolution of issues concerning their upbringing. '. . . any delay in determining the question is likely to prejudice the welfare of the child'.

The timetable of each case is regulated by a procedure known as a 'directions hearing' or 'preliminary hearing'. One purpose of the preliminary hearing is to sort out who is, or should be, a party to the proceedings and who should have notice of the proceedings. The court must ensure that the technicalities of the paperwork are in order, and that service of documents and reports will be carried out. The evidence to be called is reviewed, and a timetable drawn up for preparation of evidence and its disclosure to other parties and to the guardian ad litem. The date of the hearing will also be fixed if at all possible. The directions given will carry the force of a court order, and failure to comply will be viewed seriously by the court.

If instructed to prepare a report for court, it would be wise to consider the timetable thoroughly, ensuring that any factors in reports or assessments to be undertaken, which may cause delay, are clearly stated in advance and can be taken into account by the court when giving directions. Directions may govern the venue for a medical or social work assessment, those present, who will carry out the work, and those to whom the results shall be given. A list of 'dates to avoid' provided for court at the directions hearing will enable the case to be listed on dates convenient for witnesses. If called as a witness or asked for a report for the court, prepare a timetable straightaway for the work to be done and a list of dates when unavailable to attend court. With this information, the court can avoid unnecessary adjournments.

CONCURRENT POWERS

The Act creates a new three-tiered court comprising the High Court, county court and magistrates' court, each with concurrent jurisdiction, enabling cases to move up and down the levels as appropriate. (See Figure 1.2 for the range of powers now available under the Act in family proceedings.)

THE CHILD IS A PERSON, NOT AN OBJECT OF CONCERN

The ethos of the Act is to listen to the child's wishes and feelings, and to treat children with respect as individuals. In the past, attitudes have been paternalistic and intervention has often been with little regard to the child's expressed wishes. Children of sufficient maturity should be consulted on issues such as placements, reviews and long-term planning [1].

THE WELFARE OF THE CHILD IS THE COURT'S PARAMOUNT CONSIDERATION

Bearing in mind that the child's welfare is the court's paramount consideration, it is vital that reliable methods are used to ascertain what will be in the best interests of the child. In public law, the person who will most often advise the court on this is the guardian ad litem, an independent adviser (usually with social work training or experience) appointed by the court for this purpose [2]. In private law, the adviser will normally be the court welfare officer. The court has power to request a welfare report to be prepared on any case it considers appropriate [3].

Guardians are required to interview all those who may be able to give relevant information about the child's life and circumstances, and to interview the child. They have access to all social work files and records, and may seek additional information in order to advise the court [4]. They may request access to medical or psychiatric records of the child or of others involved in the child's life. Consent for disclosure of information is an important issue which is discussed further in Chapter 10.

WELFARE CHECKLIST

To guide the court's thinking, the Act contains a checklist of factors to which the court shall have particular regard (s 1(3)):

'(a) the ascertainable wishes and feelings of the child concerned (considered in the light of his age and understanding);
(b) his physical, emotional and educational needs;
(c) the likely effect on him of any change in his circumstances;
(d) his age, sex, background and any characteristics of his which the court considers relevant;
(e) any harm which he has suffered or is at risk of suffering;
(f) how capable each of his parents, and any other person in relation to whom the court considers the question to be relevant, is of meeting his needs;
(g) the range of powers available to the court [see Figure 1.2] under this Act in the proceedings in question.'

Interestingly, the court does not have to consider the items on the checklist in all cases. It is compulsory to consider these factors in applications to make, vary or discharge a residence, contact, prohibited steps or specific issue order if the application is opposed; or in care, s 34 contact or supervision proceedings, even if unopposed (see Figure 1.1).

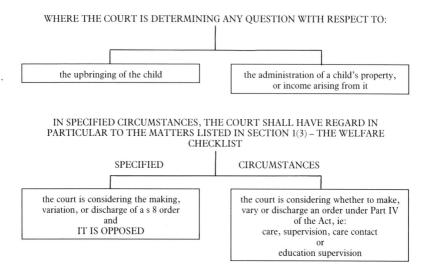

Figure 1.1 The Welfare of the Child shall be the Court's Paramount Consideration

NON-INTERVENTION

Whereas it may seem odd that it is not compulsory to consider the checklist in all cases, this does reflect another underlying principle upon which the Act is based. This is that children should be brought up by their parents or wider family without interference by the State unless they are placed at risk; and if they do have to be away from home, family links should be maintained [5]. The court will need to be alert to any unusual circumstances or factors causing concern in cases between individuals about the care or upbringing of a child, even if the parties themselves are in agreement about the application they are making to the court. In furtherance of the non-intervention principle, the court is directed, when considering making an order, not to make an order unless it considers that doing so would be better for the child than making no order at all [6].

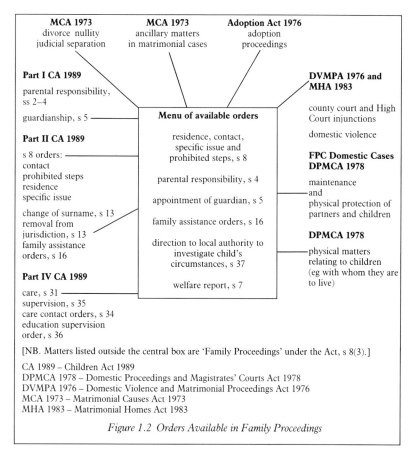

MCA 1973
divorce nullity
judicial separation

MCA 1973
ancillary matters
in matrimonial cases

Adoption Act 1976
adoption
proceedings

Part I CA 1989

parental responsibility,
ss 2–4

guardianship, s 5

Part II CA 1989

s 8 orders:
contact
prohibited steps
residence
specific issue

change of surname, s 13
removal from
jurisdiction, s 13
family assistance
orders, s 16

Part IV CA 1989

care, s 31
supervision, s 35
care contact orders, s 34
education supervision
order, s 36

Menu of available orders

residence, contact,
specific issue and
prohibited steps, s 8

parental responsibility, s 4

appointment of guardian, s 5

family assistance orders, s 16

direction to local authority to
investigate child's
circumstances, s 37

welfare report, s 7

DVMPA 1976 and MHA 1983

county court and High
Court injunctions

domestic violence

FPC Domestic Cases DPMCA 1978

maintenance
and
physical protection of
partners and children

DPMCA 1978

physical matters
relating to children
(eg with whom they are
to live)

[NB. Matters listed outside the central box are 'Family Proceedings' under the Act, s 8(3).]

CA 1989 – Children Act 1989
DPMCA 1978 – Domestic Proceedings and Magistrates' Courts Act 1978
DVMPA 1976 – Domestic Violence and Matrimonial Proceedings Act 1976
MCA 1973 – Matrimonial Causes Act 1973
MHA 1983 – Matrimonial Homes Act 1983

Figure 1.2 Orders Available in Family Proceedings

REFERENCES

1. *Principles and Practice in Regulations and Guidance* (HMSO 1989) paras 1, 19, 20, and 25; Review of Children's Cases Regulations 1991, SI 1991/895, para 7
2. Children Act 1989, s 41; Family Proceedings Courts (Children Act 1989) Rules 1991, SI 1991/1395, r 10 (for magistrates' courts); Family Proceedings Rules 1991, SI 1991/1247, r 4.10 (for High Court and county courts)
3. Children Act 1989, s 7
4. Ibid, s 42; Family Proceedings Courts (Children Act 1989) Rules 1991, SI 1991/1395, r 11 (for magistrates' courts); Family Proceedings Rules 1991, SI 1991/1247, r 4.11 (for High Court and county courts)
5. *Principles and Practice in Regulations and Guidance* (HMSO, 1989) paras 5, 7, 8–9, 11, 12–16
6. Children Act 1989, s 1(5)

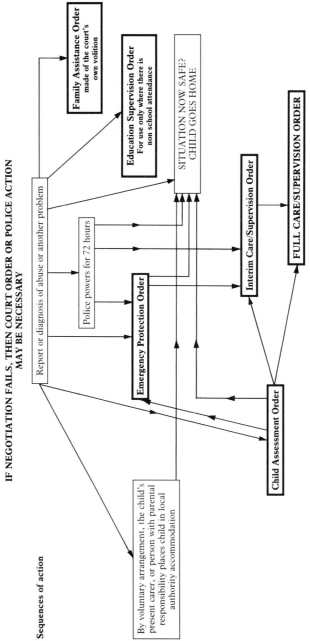

FIRST NEGOTIATE AND TRY TO AGREE SOLUTION WITH FAMILY AND CHILD
COULD CHILD STAY WITHIN FAMILY WITH INPUT OF RESOURCES?

**IF NEGOTIATION FAILS, THEN COURT ORDER OR POLICE ACTION
MAY BE NECESSARY**

Sequences of action

Report or diagnosis of abuse or another problem

Family Assistance Order
made of the court's
own volition

Education Supervision Order
For use only where there is
non school attendance

SITUATION NOW SAFE?
CHILD GOES HOME

Police powers for 72 hours

Emergency Protection Order

Interim Care/Supervision Order

FULL CARE/SUPERVISION ORDER

Child Assessment Order

By voluntary arrangement, the child's
present carer, or person with parental
responsibility places child in local
authority accommodation

Key: ☐ = COURT ORDERS

Figure 1.3 Legal Procedures to Protect Children

Chapter 2

PARENTAL RESPONSIBILITY

Many people are still unaware that on the day that the Act came into force, 14 October 1991, the legal status of all parents changed. The Act creates a new concept, 'parental responsibility', which now affects all parents in varying ways, changing many existing parental rights and powers. All those who are involved in work with children and their families, or who are themselves parents, need to know of these changes. Non-parents may also have, or acquire, parental responsibility for children. More of this later.

WHAT IS PARENTAL RESPONSIBILITY?

Formerly, parenting was, like marriage, described by one lawyer as 'a bundle of rights and duties' and the rights of children were perceived often in a negative way – the right not to be ill-treated, or the right not to be neglected. Speaking about the underlying principles of the Act it was said by one High Court judge that 'Children are people, and not objects of concern', and the Act reflects this by creating many positive rights for children, ensuring that children are respected as individuals in their own right, and that a child's wishes and feelings are not only heard but also taken into account.

Parental responsibility is defined in s 3(1) of the Act as:

'. . . all the rights, duties, powers, responsibilities and authority which by law a parent of a child has in relation to the child and his property.'

These rights and duties are not listed specifically. The rights of a child and the duties of a parent may change at various stages in a child's life to meet differing needs and circumstances. Childhood could be called a state of steadily increasing ability, and it will be apparent that as a child matures in chronological age, education and understanding, that child will be able to make increasingly important decisions on medical and other matters. This was the principle established in the well-known case of *Gillick* [1] which concerned the issue of whether a health authority could give contraceptive advice to a child under the age of 16 without the consent of her parent. It was decided that a parent could not prevent doctors giving medical advice or treatment where the child was mature enough to consent herself. For more about the legal issues around *Gillick*, and a child's ability to give medical consent, see Chapter 10.

There are, of course, other statutory provisions which impose specific duties on parents or limit their actions in some way. A parent who fails, for example to obtain essential medical assistance for her child, commits an offence [2]. Parents also have a duty under the Education Acts to ensure that their children receive adequate full-time education suited to the child's needs, aptitude and ability.

The Act gives a general power to those who have the care of a child, but who do not have parental responsibility, to do what is reasonable in all the circumstances to safeguard and promote the welfare of the child [3]. This is an enabling section for those who need to do something (for example, take a child to a doctor) but who do not have any legal rights or duties in relation to that child. It would give some power, for example to a neighbour who is babysitting for a child who is taken ill and needs urgent medical attention, and whose parents are unavailable. It would be good to think that there is a parallel positive duty to safeguard and promote the welfare of a child implied in respect of all those who actually have parental responsibility, but there is, in fact, no specific provision in the Act to this effect.

Parental responsibility is not capable of being transferred or surrendered. A parent with parental responsibility can, however, arrange for someone else to take over particular responsibilities [4]. An obvious example would be for a parent to arrange for someone else to look after her child while she is away at work or on holiday.

More than one person may have parental responsibility for the same child at the same time [5]. There is no duty under the Act for one person with parental responsibility to consult anyone else with parental responsibility before acting [6]. If there is a dispute between those with parental responsibility for a child as far as the exercise of that responsibility is concerned, they will have to resolve it by negotiation, and if attempts at peaceful resolution fail, they will have to apply to the court for a 'specific issue' order under s 8 to resolve their differences.

People other than the parents of children may also acquire parental responsibility for them. For example, if children go into statutory care, the local authority will also acquire parental responsibility, or if a grandmother obtains a residence order from the court stating that her grandchildren should live with her, she may acquire parental responsibility for them along with the order. In these circumstances, parental responsibility will be shared by all, and not lost to anyone. A local authority is able to limit the exercise of parental responsibility by a child's parents while it holds a care order. The grandmother described above would have to resolve differences of opinion with the parents by negotiation, or by application for a specific issue order or prohibited steps order if necessary.

WHO HAS PARENTAL RESPONSIBILITY?

Those who Automatically have Parental Responsibility on the Birth of the Child

Most parents acquire parental responsibility for the children born to them. They will never lose it during their lifetime unless their child is adopted. Adoption is therefore the only circumstance in which they will lose parental responsibility for their children. They may share it in ways such as those described above; if their children go into statutory care, for example, or the making of a residence order to another person; but, short of adoption, they will not lose it.

Married parents

The Act provides that a child's mother and father, if married to each other at the time of the child's conception or birth will both, automatically, have parental responsibility for the child. This principle is extended [7] to include the natural parents of a child who although unmarried at the time of the child's conception or birth subsequently marry each other, those children who are otherwise treated in law as legitimate, and those children who are adopted under the Adoption Act 1976.

For some legal and medical purposes, the time of birth may be relevant. The time of birth is deemed to extend back to the date of the insemination resulting in the birth; or, where there was no such insemination (as in in vitro fertilisation), the date of conception. This provision of the Act would therefore apply to a child whose parents divorce between the date of insemination and birth.

A father is no longer, automatically, the legal guardian of his legitimate child [8], and formerly married parents will share the parental responsibility of their children even after a divorce, although court orders under s 8 of the Act may govern particular aspects of their child's upbringing if they fail to agree on issues of parenting.

Unmarried mothers

The Act provides [9] that:

'Where a child's father and mother were not married to each other at the time of the birth –

(a) the mother shall have parental responsibility for the child;'

The mother alone, therefore, acquires full parental responsibility, automatically, at the time of the child's birth. The child's father has no parental responsibility automatically, even if he accepts his parenthood and the child is registered in his name, but he can acquire it, by agreement with the mother, by court order, or by marrying the mother.

Acquisition of Parental Responsibility

It will be clear from the earlier paragraphs that the natural father of a child (sometimes called the 'putative father' in the old terminology), and the person who becomes a step-parent of a child, will have no automatic parental responsibility for that child. The Act provides various ways in which parental responsibility may be acquired, with special provisions for its acquisition by the child's natural father.

The natural father of a child, if he is not married to the mother of the child in question (although he may, of course, be a married man), may acquire parental responsibility under the Act, either by court order or by entering into a written agreement with the mother of the child. The right to apply for a court order to gain legal rights in relation to the child of an unmarried relationship was originally introduced in the Family Law Reform Act 1987, recognising for the first time a parental role, short of custody, for unmarried fathers. The idea of a formal 'parental responsibility agreement' which can be signed and witnessed at very little cost and trouble between unmarried parents is new, and recognises the fact that something approaching one-third of children are born now to unmarried parents, who are often in a long-term relationship but who do not wish to marry.

The required form for a parental responsibility agreement is set out in a Statutory Instrument [10]. (It costs £1.00 from HMSO.) The form must be completed, then signed and dated by both the mother and the father of the child, and their signatures witnessed. There is no requirement that they have to complete the form together, provided that their signatures are duly witnessed. All that then has to be done is to send the completed form, with two copies, to the Principal Registry of the Family Division of the High Court. An officer of the Principal Registry will seal the copies and return one each to the mother and father. The Principal Registry will retain the original, and a record of the parental responsibility agreement will be available for inspection at the Principal Registry during office hours. (Copies are available upon written request and payment of a £5.00 fee.)

It will be obvious that these forms do not have a built-in lie detector. If a man is led to believe that he is the father of a child, and as a consequence agrees with the child's mother that he will have parental responsibility but later discovers that he is not the father, he will be in much the same position as a married man who believes he is the father of a child of the marriage but is told, perhaps in a moment of anger, that he is not in fact the father of that child. In the event of a dispute over parental responsibility, both parents may have to resort to litigation and possibly prove or disprove paternity by blood tests in order to sort out the ensuing muddle.

Parental responsibility agreements and parental responsibility orders may be brought to an end by the court on the application by any person with parental responsibility for the child, or by the child himself with leave of the court, provided that he has sufficient understanding to make the application.

Other people may acquire parental responsibility under the Act:

(a) a guardian;
(b) a person obtaining a residence order;
(c) a local authority named in a care order; and
(d) an applicant granted an emergency protection order, for the duration of the order.

WHAT DOES PARENTAL RESPONSIBILITY ALLOW ONE TO DO?

Those with parental responsibility for a child may make decisions on all major issues, including the child's schooling, day-to-day care, residence, maintenance and medical care, subject to certain legal safeguards, and the power of an older child to make his own decisions (see Chapter 10).

Where more than one person has parental responsibility for a child, each may act alone in meeting that responsibility unless the consent of more than one person is required under current law (for example, subject to some exceptions, married parents are both required to give consent to the marriage of their child who is under the age of 18).

The fact that a person has parental responsibility for a child does not entitle that person to use it to flout any order made under the Act [11]. If the court has made a residence order specifying that the child shall live with a named person, someone else with parental responsibility may not remove the child from the person with whom they live under that court order.

An emergency protection order or a care order gives parental responsibility to the applicant, usually the local authority. To protect the child, the local authority may restrict the use of parental responsibility by others during the subsistence of the order. The parents will not lose their parental responsibility but its use may be curtailed.

The fact that a person does, or does not, have parental responsibility will not affect any statutory obligation which that person may have in respect of the child. This includes the statutory duty to maintain the child. Neither does it affect any rights in relation to the child's property [12]. In the same way, a child's right to inherit following the death of another person is unaffected by the incidence of parental responsibility.

PARENTAL RESPONSIBILITY AND MEDICAL RECORDS

The format of medical records for children and their families should now change to take parental responsibility into account; many existing procedures must alter, particularly those for obtaining consent for the medical or psychiatric examination, assessment and treatment of children. See Chapter 10 for further discussion.

Parental Responsibility Agreement

Date Recorded

Section 4(1)(b)   The Children Act 1989

▶ Please use black ink.

▶ The making of this agreement will seriously affect the legal position of both parents.
   You should both seek legal advice before completing this form.

▶ If there is more than one child, you should fill in a separate form for each child.

THE ■■ CHILDREN ■■ ACT

This is a parental responsibility agreement between

the child's mother

> Name
>
> Address

and

the child's father

> Name
>
> Address

We agree that the father of the child named below should have parental responsibility for [him] [her] in addition to the mother.

Name	Boy/Girl	Date of birth	Date of 18th birthday

Ending of the agreement

Once a parental responsibility agreement has been made it can only end:

- by an order of the court made on application of any person who has parental responsibility for the child.
- by an order of the court made on the application of the child with leave of the court.
- when the child reaches the age of 18.

Signed (**mother**)		Date	
Signature **of witness**		Date	
Signed (**father**)		Date	
Signature **of witness**		Date	

This agreement will not take effect until this form has been filed with the Principal Registry of the Family Division. Once this form has been completed and signed please take or send it and two copies to :

> The Principal Registry of the Family Division
>
> Somerset House
>
> Strand
>
> London WC2R 1LP

THE ■■ CHILDREN ■■ ACT

JCHA1 pra

JORDANS

REFERENCES

1. *Gillick v West Norfolk & Wisbech Area Health Authority* [1986] AC 112, [1986] 1 FLR 224, discussed in Chapter 10
2. Children and Young Persons Act 1933, s 1
3. Children Act 1989, s 3(5)
4. Ibid, s 2(9)–(11)
5. Ibid, s 2(6)
6. Ibid, s 2(7) and (8)
7. Family Law Reform Act 1987
8. Children Act 1989, s 2(4)
9. Ibid, s 2(1)
10. SI 1991/1478 (ISBN 0 11 014478 3)
11. Children Act 1989, s 2(8)
12. Ibid, s 3(4)

Chapter 3

RESIDENCE AND CONTACT ORDERS

INTRODUCTION

The Act creates, in s 8, four completely new types of order: residence order, contact order, specific issue order and prohibited steps order. These new orders are intended to be used mainly in circumstances where individuals cannot reach a negotiated agreement, or cannot, for whatever reason, co-operate in the upbringing of a child. The court will always operate the principle in s 1(5) of the Act that it shall not make any order unless it considers that doing so would be better for the child than making no order at all.

The welfare of the child is of paramount importance and the principle that delay is likely to prejudice the welfare of the child will apply in making residence and contact orders. The court has power to make any additional directions and conditions as appropriate. In any family proceedings in which a question arises as to the welfare of any child, these orders may also be made of the court's own volition even though no application has been made. In theory, therefore, this could perhaps be extended to cover the sibling of a child in respect of whom family proceedings were brought, if a question of the welfare of that child arose and the court feels that an order is necessary in the child's interests.

(This chapter covers residence and contact orders; Chapter 4 covers specific issue and prohibited steps orders.)

LOCAL AUTHORITY MAY NOT USE RESIDENCE OR SECTION 8 CONTACT ORDERS

Sometimes a local authority can make use of orders available under the Act, but a local authority may *not* apply for a residence order or a contact order under s 8 of the Act, and no court may make such an order in favour of a local authority. There are provisions for contact with a child in care under Part IV of the Act, and another, entirely separate order is available under s 34, colloquially called the 'care contact order' to distinguish it from a s 8 contact order.

LIMITATIONS FOR CHILDREN IN STATUTORY CARE OF LOCAL AUTHORITY

The only order under s 8 which can be made in respect of a child in statutory care is a residence order. If this is made, it must necessarily be in favour of someone other than the local authority and it will then automatically discharge the care order. The court will have considered the effect of making the residence order before making its decision.

RESIDENCE ORDERS

Definition

A residence order is an order which determines with whom the child is to live. Note that it specifies the person with whom the child will live. However, the place at which the child will live could be settled by directions in the order.

Scope of the Order

This new, residence order replaces the old familiar custody, and care and control orders. The intention of the legislators was that it should give the court more flexibility in the exercise of its powers, and also that it should not be sought automatically as part of a divorce package, or separation agreement, but that it should be available as and when necessary. Its use is not limited to difficulties between couples over the residence of their children, but it may be sought by anyone who wishes to care for a particular child in their home, an obvious example being grandparents.

It is not restricted to one applicant. A residence order may be made in favour of more than one person where it is in the interests of the child to do so. A shared residence order would accommodate the shared care arrangements typical of many households where the partners have decided to live apart. Examples would be an order for a child to live with the mother during the school term-time and with the father during the school holidays; or with a grandmother during the week and with the father at weekends.

Residence Orders and Parental Responsibility

It is logical that the person with whom a child lives will need to have some legal recognition of his or her decision-making powers in respect of the child. That person may need to have all the legal rights, responsibilities and duties which together comprise 'parental responsibility' (discussed in Chapter 2). The court may give parental responsibility, along with a residence order, and it will subsist for as long as the residence order lasts.

There is a special exception in the case of an unmarried father of a child who gains a residence order, and along with it parental responsibility that he did not have before (ie he had not already acquired it by agreement or court order). In this case, the father will retain the parental responsibility until it is removed from him by the court, even if the residence order ceases.

It was the intention of the legislation, and made clear in the *Guidance* later published [1] that both parents should have a continuing role to play in the lives of their children wherever possible.

Existing parental responsibility is unaffected by the making of a residence order. If, for example, the parents of a child both have parental responsibility, and a residence order is made to a grandmother, she may acquire parental responsibility with her residence order, and will share it with the child's parents or anyone else who has it [2].

Parental responsibility may be exercised by each person who has it, completely independently of the others who also have it, without any duty to consult each other [3], but not in contravention of any court order or statutory requirement [4]. This is, it seems, a really practical test of the principles of co-operation and negotiation, but could lead to more, rather than less litigation.

Special Rights/Powers/Limitations under Residence Orders

(a) Where a person who is not the child's parent or guardian acquires a residence order for that child, that person may not consent to the child's adoption, nor to an order freeing the child for adoption, nor may that person appoint a guardian for the child [5]. If a guardian is needed, the court has power to appoint one under s 5.

(b) While a residence order is in force, the surname of the child may not be changed without the written consent of every person who has parental responsibility for the child, or an order of the court [6].

(c) While a residence order is in force, the child subject to the order may not be taken out of the UK without the written consent of every person who has parental responsibility for the child, or an order of the court [7]. To get around this problem the court may grant general leave or leave limited for specified purposes when making the residence order.

But a special exception . . .

(d) A residence order carries with it the right for the person in whose favour the order is made to take a child out of the United Kingdom for a period of up to one month without having to obtain the written consent of all those with parental responsibility [8].

The Act [9] amends the Child Abduction Act 1984 to take account of the new residence orders, and other provisions of the Act. In all other circumstances, there will be an offence committed under the Child Abduction Act 1984 if the consents required by that Act to take a child abroad are not properly obtained.

Who can Apply for a Residence Order?

A parent (mother or father, whether married or not) or a guardian of a child may apply as of right.

There are special additional categories of people who may also apply as of right for residence or contact orders [10]:

(a) the parties to a marriage of whom the child is a 'child of the family' (meaning accepted by the partners as a child of the family);

(b) anyone with whom the child has lived for at least three years;

(c) those having the consent of anyone with an existing residence order;

(d) those having the consent of the local authority if the child is in care;

(e) those who have the consent of all those who have parental responsibility for the child.

Any other person may apply for a residence order provided that they first obtain the leave of the court to do so. The court acts as a 'gatekeeper' to stop unnecessary or repeated applications that may not be in the child's best interests. Members of the child's wider family, such as grandparents, would be likely to obtain leave unless there were circumstances making it contrary to the child's interests for an application to be made.

A child with sufficient understanding may apply for a residence order to go and live with a named person, with leave of the court.

There are restrictions on applications made by those who are or have been local authority foster-parents to the child in the previous six months [11].

When considering an application for leave to seek a residence order, the court must consider several matters including the risk of disruption to the child, and the applicant's connection with the child [12].

Duration of Residence Orders

Residence orders will normally last only until the child reaches the age of 16. After that, a child is usually mature enough to make decisions about where he wants to live. In exceptional circumstances, the order may be extended until the child reaches the age of 18, perhaps where a child has learning disabilities or is unable for any reason to be independent in decision-making, or in need of continuing care [13].

CONTACT ORDERS

Definition

A contact order is an order requiring the person with whom a child lives, or is to live, to allow that child to visit or stay with the person named in the order, or for that person and the child to have contact with each other. The order is empowering. To prevent contact, a prohibited steps order may be used and any delay in determining the question will be deemed to be prejudicial to the child's interests.

Scope of the Order

A contact order is wide. Contact is envisaged as including anything from visits to letters, tape recordings, video recordings, parcels, telephone calls, and birthday or other celebratory presents. Contact may be direct or indirect and supervised where necessary. The court has wide power to regulate contact if necessary by specific directions or conditions, or to leave the details such as means, location, frequency and duration of contact to the respective parties to negotiate themselves. The principles of non-intervention will apply, and no order will be made unless it is in the child's interests to do so.

Who can Apply for a Contact Order?

The child's parents (mother or father whether married or not), and any person with a residence order in their favour with respect to the child may apply as of right. There are special additional categories of people who may also apply, as of right, for residence or contact orders (for the complete list please refer to 'who can apply for a residence order?' above.

Anyone else can apply with the leave of the court, and the principles of the child's welfare, avoidance of delay and non-intervention will apply in making a decision, together with other matters to which the court must have regard [12].

Duration of Contact Orders

Contact orders will normally be worded to remain in force until the child reaches the age of 16, or an earlier date. After that, a child is usually mature enough to make decisions about those with whom he wants contact. In exceptional circumstances, the order may be extended until the child reaches the age of 18, perhaps where a child has learning disabilities or is unable for any reason to be independent in decision-making, or in need of continuing protection or care [14].

Contact orders may be varied or terminated through an application by any of the parties to the original order, the person named in the order, or the child.

The *Guidance* [15] makes a stand for the rights of parents to have contact with their children, particularly fathers:

'Family links should be actively maintained through visits and other forms of contact. Both parents are important, even if one of them is no longer in the family home and fathers should not be overlooked or marginalised.'

CONTACT WITH CHILDREN IN STATUTORY CARE

The Act and the *Guidance* around it emphasise the importance of maintaining continuity of a child's existing relationships. The *Guidance* [16] recognises that attachments should be respected, sustained and developed. The Act therefore creates a new contact order under s 34 for children who are in the care of a local authority under a court order. For further information please refer to Chapter 8 on care and supervision orders. Those children who are in local authority accommodation on a voluntary basis (formerly called 'voluntary care') will be subject to the provisions of s 8 of the Act as described above.

REFERENCES

1. *Principles and Practice in Regulations and Guidance* (HMSO, 1989), para 14
2. Children Act 1989, s 2(6)–(8)
3. Ibid, s 2(7)
4. Ibid, s 2(8)
5. Ibid, s 12(2) and (3)
6. Ibid, s 13(1)(a)
7. Ibid, s 13(1)(b)
8. Ibid, s 13(2) and (3)
9. Ibid, Sch 12, paras 37–40
10. Ibid, s 10(5)
11. Ibid, s 9(3) and (4)
12. Ibid, s 10(9)
13. Ibid, s 91(10) and (11)
14. Ibid, s 91(10) and (11)
15. *Principles and Practice in Regulations and Guidance* (HMSO, 1989), para 14
16. Ibid, para 15

Chapter 4

SPECIFIC ISSUE AND PROHIBITED STEPS ORDERS

Specific issue and prohibited steps orders are the other two new family proceedings orders created by s 8 of the Act. They may be made in conjunction with other orders under the Act, subject only to the needs of each individual case, and the specific limitations on the scope of each order imposed by the Act itself.

To encourage maximum flexibility for the courts, s 8 orders may be made of the court's own volition during the course of family proceedings, without any application for that particular order having been made. Those who go to court having applied for one order, say, residence, could therefore find themselves going home with an additional order or even something completely different! It should be remembered that the court may make any order it feels appropriate or no order at all as is consistent with the best interests of the child. Those who work with children and families in these circumstances must bear in mind the court's wide range of powers, and advise accordingly (see Figure 1.2).

In many ways, specific issue and prohibited steps orders are complementary to each other, while fulfilling opposite functions. The specific issue order is designed to sort out a situation where those who have the care of a child, are interested in the child's welfare, or have parental responsibility for a child, disagree about the exercise of a particular aspect of parental responsibility and they are unable to reach an agreement or compromise. A prohibited steps order is available to prevent the exercise of parental responsibility in a particular way without the consent of the court. In basic terms, one order directs 'go and do it this way' (specific issue) while the other forbids 'don't do it without permission' (prohibited steps).

Both of these orders are available to local authorities in that they may apply for the order in relation to a child in whose welfare they are interested, but these orders may *not* be made in relation to a child who is subject to a care order.

In the past, wardship would often have been used to resolve serious cases involving disagreements over a child's upbringing, but under the Act the power of the High Court is available without the necessity for wardship. The High Court is the upper level of 'the court' [1] which may make the full range of orders available under the Act, therefore specific issue or prohibited steps orders may be sought at any level – cases being transferred up or down within the tiers of the court as appropriate.

Parliament intended the court to have wide powers. Orders should be readily available without cumbersome procedures. Wardship has now been curtailed, and is only available to local authorities in very limited circumstances [2]. The introduction of the specific issue and prohibited steps orders was intended to reduce the use of wardship generally. Wardship uses up considerable court time and, because it involves a continuing duty for the High Court to oversee the warded child's upbringing, involves considerable administration. Important steps in every ward's life must first be sanctioned by the court.

A local authority can apply, just as any other individual, with the leave of the court, for a specific issue or prohibited steps order, and these orders may be invoked when a child needs particular medical treatment and parent(s) are refusing it (specific issue); or where it is not considered to be in a child's medical or psychological interests to undergo a particular procedure that parents wish to impose upon the child (pro-hibited steps). Local authorities may not use specific issue or prohibited steps as a back-door way to obtain the care or supervision of a child, to accommodate a child, or to gain parental responsibility. These orders were not designed for this purpose, and the only route into care is via a properly proved application to the court for a care order under the Act.

SPECIFIC ISSUE ORDERS

Definition

'. . . an order giving directions for the purpose of determining a specific question which has arisen, or which may arise, in connection with any aspect of parental responsibility for a child.' [3]

Scope of the Order

The *Guidance* [4] says that:

'The aim is not to give one parent or the other a general "right" to make decisions about a particular aspect of the child's upbringing, for example his education or medical treatment, but rather to enable a particular dispute over such a matter to be resolved by the court, including the giving of detailed directions where necessary.'

It will be clear that a specific issue order cannot be used generally, but that it would be useful where a problem involving, for example medical treatment or schooling arises, which the parents cannot resolve amicably.

As has been seen above, local authorities may make use of this order where a child is not in statutory care, and it may prove useful where a child is being looked after by the authority on a voluntary basis and needs a specific course of medical treatment and the child's parents cannot be contacted.

The *Guidance* [4] says of this situation, rather laconically:

'If, in all the circumstances of the case, the decision is likely to cause controversy at some future date, the local authority should seek a section 8 specific issue order.'

An obvious example of a potentially controversial situation is where a blood transfusion is considered medically necessary, and either child or parents are known to hold religious beliefs that would not permit such treatment. One religious organisation has amassed medical and legal materials to assist members and their legal advisers, with access to a directory of consultants who understand the special needs of those who wish to have operations without the use of homologous blood [5]. Attempts by local authorities and/or hospital authorities to override parental requests for alternative non-blood medical management may well be opposed, and, in these circumstances, a specific issue order may be sought as an emergency application to enable the court to resolve the issues raised.

In emergencies, the court has power to reduce notice or to waive notice altogether, and there is a rota in each area of justices and judges who are on duty in out-of-court hours who may be contacted by telephone. Hospitals and surgeries should have emergency court numbers available for reference.

In other circumstances, or in an absolute emergency where an application for specific issue for some reason is impossible, the doctor may decide to act in accordance with the normal medical ethics of practice in the event of emergencies involving adults or children where the patient is unable to give consent themselves [6].

On a practical level, if there is any concern or doubt at all about the legal position regarding a child in any specific case, the legal department of the local authority should be consulted and will be able to advise. There is also a NHS booklet of guidance for health practitioners [7], however, unfortunately, the current edition does not fully address the problems raised by parental responsibility and medical consent, nor the provisions of the Act. The authors understand that it may soon be revised (see Chapter 10 for discussion of recent cases).

Who may Apply for a Specific Issue Order?

Parents (mother and father, whether married to each other or not), guardians, and anyone who has a residence order in their favour in respect of the child, may apply for a specific issue order in relation to that child as of right. Anyone else may apply for the order, but will first need the leave of the court [8].

Duration of Specific Issue Orders

Specific issue orders may not extend beyond the child's sixteenth birthday unless the circumstances are exceptional [9]. The court may give whatever directions or conditions in the making of the order as it sees fit. The order may be varied or terminated on the application of anyone entitled to apply for the order, or the previous applicant.

PROHIBITED STEPS ORDERS

Definition

'. . . an order that no step which could be taken by a parent in meeting his parental responsibility for a child, and which is of a kind specified in the order, shall be taken by any person without the consent of the court;' [10]

Scope of the Order

A prohibited steps order is designed for one particular situation at a time. It was not intended for long-term generalised situations. Its most obvious use is to prevent one parent taking his child abroad without the necessary consents required by statute [11]. The *Guidance* suggests that it may also be used for the prevention of the child's removal from home before the court has had time to decide what other order, if any, to make [12].

Interestingly, it seems from its definition that the order may be made against anybody (not just the child's parents or those who have parental responsibility for a child) but the action which it forbids must be one that could be taken by a parent in meeting parental responsibility.

Who may Apply for a Prohibited Steps Order?

Parents – the child's mother and father, irrespective of whether they are (or were) married to each other, guardians, and anyone else who has a residence order in their favour in respect of the child – may apply as of right for a prohibited steps order in relation to that child. Anyone else, including the child, may apply for the order, but would first need the leave of the court [13].

Duration of Prohibited Steps Order

Prohibited steps orders may not extend beyond the child's sixteenth birthday unless there are exceptional circumstances. The court has a wide power to make whatever directions or conditions as it sees fit. The order may be varied or terminated by the court at the request of anyone entitled to apply for the order, or the previous applicant.

REFERENCES

1. Children Act 1989, s 92(7). See also Glossary
2. Ibid, s 100
3. Ibid, s 8(1)
4. *The Children Act 1989 Guidance and Regulations Volume 1 Court Orders*, para 2.33
5. Medico–Legal Department, Watchtower House, London NW7 1RN
6. See Chapter 10 for medical consents
7. *A Guide to Consent for Examination or Treatment* (NHS Management Executive), see Appendix 2
8. Children Act 1989, s 10

9. Ibid, s 92(10) and (11)
10. Ibid, s 8(1)
11. See Chapter 3 on residence and contact orders, pp 15–21
12. *The Children Act 1989 Guidance and Regulations Volume 1 Court Orders*, para 2.31
13. Children Act 1989, s 10

Chapter 5

EMERGENCY PROTECTION ORDERS

INTRODUCTION

Emergency protection orders supersede place of safety orders, the use of which, prior to the Act, was often criticised. The new order differs in many aspects, its function being solely to protect the child in an emergency. Checks and balances have been introduced to prevent orders being used as a device to initiate care proceedings, or to coerce supposedly non-cooperative parents. Magistrates must be scrupulous as to the grounds being met before granting an order.

WHO MAY APPLY?

Any person may apply for an order where a child is likely to suffer significant harm if he is not removed to accommodation provided by or on behalf of the applicant; or does not remain where he is being accommodated.

A local authority may also apply for an order where it is making inquiries about a child under its duty to investigate, and access to that child is urgently required and is being unreasonably prevented.

Representatives of other agencies, including those from health services or the police may apply. However, as the police have their own powers [1], health practitioners are the more likely alternative applicants.

Even so, whilst practitioners are able to apply as individuals, the most probable situation is that their evidence will be used by the local authority when the local authority is the applicant, including when the investigation is initiated by the practitioner.

Family members, or a parent, can apply for an order, but as the local authority has to be involved because of its duty to investigate, this will probably happen rarely.

SIGNIFICANT HARM

Whoever applies will have to provide the court with evidence that the child is likely to suffer significant harm. Proof that the child has suffered in the past will not be sufficient; emergency protection is from potential or current circumstances, not past dangers.

When the local authority is investigating and unable to gain access to the child, it will have to show that because inquiries are being frustrated it is not possible to establish if significant harm is occurring, or is likely to occur. In addition, the need for urgency will have to be shown.

Prediction of significant harm being the salient point, the court may accept any relevant evidence. This can include hearsay, health or social services reports, opinion, observation, or direct medical judgment.

TIMING OF THE ORDER

The applicant will have to establish urgency as it is an emergency order, having a duration of up to eight days. An extension of seven days can be granted. The emergency nature of the order will usually mean that initial applications will not be made on notice, or notice will be short.

The applicant has to show that the parents are not co-operating and removal cannot wait for care proceedings to be initiated. Emergency removal of the child will probably be traumatic and has to be weighed against the potential harm of non-removal.

The order cannot be appealed, but application for its discharge may be made after 72 hours and within eight days. Application can be made by the child, his parents, those with parental responsibility, or any person with whom the child was living immediately prior to the order.

Local authorities may not wish to apply for an extension to an order but, instead, make an application for an interim care order pending a full care hearing. As interim care orders can last for up to eight weeks while extended emergency protection orders are much shorter, parents will probably be advised to apply for a discharge of the order as early as possible after it was made. Courts will want to be satisfied that there is a very good reason for an order being extended.

CONSEQUENCES OF THE ORDER

Whoever is able to do so must comply with the order and produce the child for the applicant. The child may then be accommodated by the applicant or on their behalf, including hospitalisation. A refusal to produce the child can lead to a warrant being issued, allowing a constable to assist and, if necessary, use appropriate force. The order includes the right to search for the child in named premises and may include other children believed to be there. The police have additional powers [2] to gain entry if life and limb is believed to be threatened.

A child produced unharmed, with no likelihood of significant harm, should not be removed from his home. Where a child is removed and the situation becomes safe, the child should be returned to his home during the period of an order. Where possible and appropriate, alleged perpetrators of abuse should move out of the home so that the child can remain at home, or return to it. If the child is asleep, a parent may agree to present him to a doctor at another, more reasonable, time. A decision has to be made as to the potential danger the child will be in when assessing the reasonableness of such offers.

The applicant gains temporary parental responsibility for the duration of the order. This enables the applicant to accommodate the child and promote the child's welfare. It is not intended to be for the purpose of making long-term decisions about the child's life. Proper attention must be given to arranging contact between the child and his family. Where this is believed to be harmful, as it may be in cases of suspected sexual or emotional abuse, or particular violence, contact with specified individuals may be controlled by the court. The court should be notified of any intended denial of contact, or request for its supervision. The court may regulate the child's contact with any appropriate person or leave it to the discretion of the local authority. Refusal of contact may be contested.

THE ROLE OF MEDICAL PRACTITIONERS AND PSYCHIATRISTS

The emergency nature of the order indicates that medical examination or treatment will be likely. This may be to gain evidence for care proceedings, as well as looking to the child's immediate medical needs. Practitioners must be aware that they may be called to give evidence in any ensuing proceedings. Courts may direct that a practitioner can accompany social workers when an order is being executed. Practitioners' evidence may be required at a later date as well as tending to the child's immediate needs.

It will not always be possible for certain practitioners to be available at short notice. Hospital services will, therefore, need to be aware of potential requests for involvement. Accident and emergency departments should arrange for the duty paediatrician to see the child, or a duty psychiatrist may be required.

Courts will be concerned that the child is not abused by over-intrusive or multiple examinations. A guardian ad litem should be appointed at the earliest opportunity to advise as to the child's best interests. If parents are challenging a medical assessment, it may be agreed that their chosen practitioner is present throughout examinations.

Consent to examination can be given by the applicant as they have acquired temporary parental responsibility. Court orders, when containing directions on this matter, are binding. Courts may deny examination pending a hearing. Parents will not be able to challenge the order until 72 hours have elapsed and the local authority may wish to support any objection to parents' applications with medical evidence. The guardian would advise the court and may be able to negotiate mutually acceptable practitioners. It should be noted that the court should make directions as to medical or psychiatric intervention. If there is a failure to seek directions or they are not properly complied with, the court, as a sanction, may not allow the information to be presented in subsequent hearings [3].

A child or young person may refuse to submit to a medical or psychiatric examination or assessment. In these circumstances, a decision has to be made as to whether the child has sufficient understanding and has been properly informed. No person, including the court, is expected to cajole the child into consenting. The guardian will want to ensure that the child is fully aware of the situation and find out whether the child still refuses to consent.

Practitioners may not proceed to examine or assess a child who has given an informed refusal under the Act. A distinction should, however, be drawn between necessary medical treatment and an examination or assessment for purely forensic purposes. Unless the situation is life-threatening or very urgent, any refusal to undergo examination or assessment should be referred back to the court [4].

Practitioners should also be aware that if an application is made by a local authority for a child assessment order [5], the court may find that the circumstances warrant the making of an emergency protection order. In these circumstances, practitioners will already have arranged a timetable for assessment or treatment and should therefore be prepared.

CONCLUSION

Emergency protection orders are exactly that; they are not a device to start other proceedings. Courts are expected to be vigilant in their issuing of directions, and applications will not be rubber-stamped. It will have to be shown that the child is likely to suffer harm rather than that he has previously suffered. Where possible, the suspected perpetrators of abuse should remove themselves from the child's home to avoid such an order. Removal of the child is traumatic and can be, ironically, punitive to the child.

Practitioners are most likely to be involved at a number of levels, commonly from the earliest stages of the order. Such situations are complex and traumatic for all parties, particularly the child. Practitioners will have to integrate their medical knowledge with as sympathetic an approach as is possible. Traumatised children may need to have a clear explanation as to what is happening so that they can give informed consent.

Courts and guardians will be likely to request that practitioners supply them with reports. If the local authority is applying for an interim care order it will be asked to supply evidence. When a court directs that a child be examined or treated, a medical report is usually requested.

Although the order is an emergency measure, the court must apply the principles of the Act that the child's welfare is paramount, that the making of an order is better for the child than no order at all, and that delay is likely to prejudice his welfare. The child should return home if the situation becomes safe. The child should not be removed if, on investigation, it is found he has not been, nor is likely to be, harmed. This will often depend on medical opinion. The role of practitioners in the execution of emergency protection orders is therefore most important.

It is vital for all the disciplines involved in child protection to co-operate and communicate effectively with each other. Practitioners should always try to attend case conferences when invited [6]. The comments on race, culture and gender in Chapter 8 at p 51 apply equally here.

REFERENCES

1. Children Act 1989, s 46
2. Police and Criminal Evidence Act 1984, s 17(1)(e)
3. Family Proceedings Rules 1991, SI 1991/1247, r 4.18
4. See Chapter 10 for further discussion
5. See Chapter 8
6. See *Working Together Under the Children Act* (HMSO, 1991)

Chapter 6

POLICE PROTECTION

EXTENT OF POLICE POWERS

In an emergency, where a police officer has reasonable cause to believe that a child would otherwise be likely to suffer significant harm, the police have the power to remove that child to suitable accommodation and to keep him there; or to take such steps as are reasonable to prevent the child's removal from any hospital, or other place in which he is then being accommodated [1].

This is a most useful power. If a child is admitted to hospital or to a doctor's surgery, the police may prevent anyone removing that child. This, and the power to remove a child to police protection, do not need a court order. If there is a situation requiring immediate action, and perhaps not even time for an emergency protection order, the police may act immediately. Where called out to a difficult case, social workers or doctors may be accompanied by a police officer, who is then able to use this power.

TIME-LIMITS

This power should not be abused. It is only for urgent and serious cases, and will last only for a period of 72 hours. This should be sufficient time for the local authority to decide which, if any, court order should be sought.

WHO MUST BE INFORMED?

If a child is taken into police protection, the local authority of the area in which the child was found must be informed as soon as reasonably practicable of the steps which have been taken and the reasons for them. If the child has sufficient understanding, he must be given the same information, told of further steps which may be taken, and his wishes and feelings ascertained. The authority in whose area the child is ordinarily resident should also be told of the place where the child is being accommodated.

FURTHER ACTION AFTER IMPLEMENTATION OF POLICE PROTECTION

A designated police officer must inquire into the case.

If the child has been removed by the police to accommodation which is not a Children Act Refuge [2], or provided by the local authority, then the child should be taken to a refuge or local authority accommodation immediately.

The child's parents, those with parental responsibility for the child and anyone with whom the child was living immediately before the police protection occurred, should be informed of what has been done as soon as reasonably practicable, and also told of further steps to be taken.

Once the designated officer has completed the inquiries, the child should be released from police protection unless there is a continuing danger of significant harm. If there is a continuing danger of significant harm to the child, the designated officer may apply for an emergency protection order on behalf of the local authority for the area in which the child is ordinarily resident, whether or not that authority knows of or agrees to the application.

The designated officer acquires no parental responsibility for the child, but has power to do what is necessary for the child's welfare.

CONTACT WITH A CHILD IN POLICE PROTECTION

The designated officer or the local authority looking after the child shall allow the child's parents, those with parental responsibility for the child, and those with whom the child was living immediately before the police protection, to have reasonable contact provided that it is in the child's best interests. Those who are allowed contact with the child under a court order are also to be permitted contact while the child is in police protection, provided this is in the child's interests (see *Figure 1.3 Legal Procedures to Protect Children* for further courses of action following police protection).

REFERENCES

1. Children Act 1989, s 46
2. Ibid, s 51

Chapter 7

CARE AND SUPERVISION ORDERS

ONLY ONE ROUTE INTO CARE

The Act radically reforms the law of care and supervision. Formerly, there were a number of routes into care over and above the case of the child's development being avoidably impaired. Care orders could be made as a 'sentence' in criminal proceedings against a juvenile, in matrimonial proceedings at the instigation of the judge, and as a sanction for non-school attendance. Now there is only one way into care.

The court may make a care order only if satisfied that the grounds set out in the Act [1] are proved. The principles that the court shall not make an order unless it is in the interests of the child, and the avoidance of delay, both apply [2]. The court must also have regard to the matters listed in the welfare checklist [3].

ONLY A LOCAL AUTHORITY OR AUTHORISED PERSON MAY APPLY FOR A CARE ORDER

An 'authorised person' is, currently, an officer of the NSPCC. Only they, and a local authority may apply for care or supervision orders. If a court feels that these possibilities should be considered, it may direct a local authority to investigate a child's circumstances and report back to the court, making an application if the investigation shows that a care order is necessary or giving reasons why no application is required [4].

NEW GROUNDS FOR CARE AND SUPERVISION

The Act creates new grounds for care (s 31(2)). These are:

'(a) that the child concerned is suffering, or is likely to suffer, significant harm; and

(b) that the harm, or likelihood of harm, is attributable to –

(i) the care given to the child, or likely to be given to him if the order were not made, not being what it would be reasonable to expect a parent to give to him; or

(ii) the child's being beyond parental control.'

The flow chart below (Figure 7.1) may assist in thinking through the concept of significant harm, and assessment of the cause of any harm or likely harm identified.

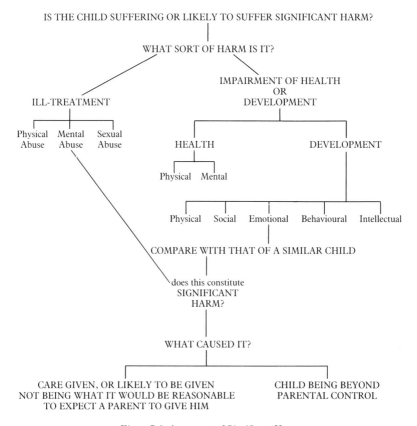

Figure 7.1 Assessment of Significant Harm

- **Harm** is defined in the Act [5] as 'ill-treatment or the impairment of health or development'.
- **Development** means physical, intellectual, emotional, social or behavioural development.
- **Health** includes physical or mental health.
- **Ill-treatment** includes sexual abuse and forms of ill-treatment which are not physical [6].

The inclusion in the legislation of sexual and emotional abuse is useful and important, as is the likelihood of significant harm in the future.

The difficulty for practitioners in these grounds is the definition of 'significant harm'. The Act [7] provides that:

> 'Where the question of whether harm suffered by a child is significant turns on the child's health or development, his health or development shall be compared with that which could reasonably be expected of a similar child.'

The court will have to compare this particular child with a notional similar child, and assess the differences. It remains to be seen how the courts will interpret this provision.

The court must not only find the existence or likelihood of significant harm but also its cause – which to form enough for a care or supervision order, must be attributable to parental care falling below a reasonable standard, or the child being beyond parental control. The test is objective, measured against a reasonable standard of parenting.

EFFECT OF CARE ORDER

The local authority acquires parental responsibility, sharing it with those who already have it in relation to the child [8]. The local authority may, however, limit the exercise by others of their parental responsibility while the care order subsists [9]. There are limits on the powers of the local authority while it has a care order. It may not change a child's religion, consent to his adoption, or appoint a guardian for the child [10]. The power of others is also limited during a care order [11]. The child's name may not be changed or the child removed from the UK without the written consent of all those with parental responsibility or leave of the court.

CONTACT WITH CHILDREN IN STATUTORY CARE

Contact with children in care used to be at the total discretion of a local authority, but now the court has control. Subject to special provisions in the Act [12], the court may make whatever order it considers appropriate in respect of contact between the child and a named person. Subject to these provisions, the local authority must allow reasonable contact with a child in care to parents, guardians, those who had a residence order in force at the time the care order was made, and those who had care of the child under a High Court order [13]. In urgent cases, for the best interests of the child, a local authority may stop contact for up to seven days only. If the local authority wishes to stop contact for more than seven days, it must apply to the court for a 'care contact order' under s 34 of the Act authorising contact to be refused to a named person. The child has the right to apply for a care contact order, and the court may make an order of its own volition when making a care order or in family proceedings for a child in care.

EFFECT OF SUPERVISION ORDER

This order places the child under the supervision of a local authority or a probation officer. The duties and powers of the supervising officer are set out in the Act [14]. Basically, it is 'to advise, assist and befriend' the child. Sanctions for non-cooperation are to apply back to the court to discharge the order and to substitute something else. Conditions may be made in supervision orders binding those responsible for the child and the child himself; and can include directions to attend activities, or live at specified places. These directions can apply for any set period, up to the duration of the order.

MEDICAL AND PSYCHIATRIC EXAMINATION AND TREATMENT UNDER SUPERVISION ORDER

The court may direct attendance for medical or psychiatric examination or, if necessary, in-patient or out-patient treatment, which a child of sufficient understanding has a right to refuse [15]. Before making these directions, the court must know that satisfactory arrangements have been, or can be, made for the treatment proposed. This implies that the practitioner(s) concerned have indicated that they agree to carry it out. If of sufficient understanding, the child's consent is also required.

If a practitioner is unwilling to continue treatment of the child, or the directions need altering because:

– the treatment should be extended beyond the period specified in the order;
– different treatment is required;
– the child is not susceptible to treatment; or
– no further treatment is required,

the practitioner must submit a written report to the supervisor, who will then have to put that report back to the court for revision of the directions [16].

EDUCATION SUPERVISION ORDERS

A care order was formerly an available sanction for failure to attend school, but now a new order has been devised for this problem, recognising that school refusal is more likely to be a family difficulty needing the co-operation of the child, the family, the education authority and the local authority [17]. Where circumstances show the appropriate grounds, proceedings for a care order may be brought.

INTERIM CARE AND SUPERVISION ORDERS/MEDICAL AND PSYCHIATRIC ASSESSMENTS

On adjourning a care or supervision application, the court has the power to make an interim order when it is satisfied that there are reasonable grounds for believing the circumstances justifying a care order exist [18]. The duration of interim orders are limited by the Act to an initial maximum of eight weeks, followed by extensions of up to four weeks each. The Act also envisages shorter interim orders [19]. The Act seeks to avoid delay in dealing with cases. Courts will not permit repeated interim orders without very good reason.

On the making of an interim order, directions may require medical or psychiatric examination or assessment of the child which, if the child is of sufficient understanding, he may refuse [20]. Directions may also be used to prevent the abuse of children by repeated examinations for forensic or other purposes, by forbidding examinations or assessments unless otherwise directed [21].

DURATION OF CARE AND SUPERVISION ORDERS

No care order may be made for a child over the age of 17, or 16 if married [22].

Supervision orders last for one year at a time (unless discharged earlier), with the possibility of extensions up to a maximum of three years.

REFERENCES

 1. Children Act 1989, s 31
 2. See Chapter 1
 3. See Chapter 1, and the welfare checklist p 3
 4. Children Act 1989, s 37
 5. Ibid, s 31(9)
 6. Ibid, s 31(9)
 7. Ibid, s 31(10)
 8. See Chapter 2
 9. Children Act 1989, s 33(3)
10. Ibid, s 33(6)
11. Ibid, s 33(7)
12. Ibid, s 34(1)–(7)
13. Ibid, s 34
14. Ibid, s 31, s 35 and Sch 3
15. Ibid, Sch 3, paras 4 and 5
16. Ibid, Sch 3, para 5(6)–(7)
17. Ibid, s 36
18. Ibid, s 38(2)
19. Ibid, s 38(4) and (5)
20. Ibid, s 38(6) and see Chapter 10
21. Ibid, s 38(7)
22. Ibid, s 31(3)

Chapter 8

CHILD ASSESSMENT ORDERS

INTRODUCTION

The local authority has a duty to investigate when it is believed that a child is suffering significant harm or is likely to do so [1].

The Act brings together, in Part V, the legal framework for child protection (see Figure 1.3). This contains the necessary checks and balances for parents and others with a proper interest in the child, to challenge actions before the court.

When it is believed that a child may be suffering significant harm, for any reason, including abuse or neglect, but is not in immediate danger, an assessment should be made. If the parents, or those responsible for the child, refuse to allow such an assessment to take place, the local authority, or properly authorised person (eg the NSPCC), may apply to the court for a child assessment order [2].

This is less interventionist than an emergency protection order. The child is not necessarily removed to provide protection. Moreover, access to the child is granted to those with the appropriate knowledge and qualifications so that they can assess the child's current medical and social status, subsequently making recommendations.

The child assessment order did not exist in any previous legislation. Its inclusion is mainly due to the recommendation by the report into the death of Kimberley Carlile [3]. Previously, if it was believed that a child needed to be assessed, a variety of legal interventions might, possibly, have taken place. Often, in practice, the local authority resorted to wardship in the High Court with all the incumbent complications of that process.

It was felt in establishing the child assessment order, that the courts, if they had to intervene, should have more authority than purely requiring that the child be produced. Production of a child does not necessarily ensure that an assessment of that child takes place, only that he is seen. A variety of inquiries into child deaths had established that purely being seen is no indication of whether a child is suffering, or likely to suffer, significant harm, and therefore offers no guarantee of potential protection. Children in this situation need to be medically and socially assessed so that opinions can be appropriately informed and modified. If firm evidence of significant harm already exists, a child assessment order should not be applied for as such evidence can be used to apply for a variety of other protective orders, either on an emergency, interim or longer-term basis. The child assessment order exists for occasions when the lack of such information would in itself undermine any legal action which might be thought to be appropriate.

WHEN IS AN APPLICATION MADE?

Original concern about a child may be expressed by one or any number of individuals who have contact with the child and/or his family. They may be neighbours or relatives, for example, whose knowledge of a particular situation leads them to approach various agencies, who then have a responsibility to launch an investigation. Equally, a practitioner who is involved with a family may believe that a child is at risk of abuse or neglect and so implement the child protection procedures. This could be a health visitor, general practitioner, school nurse, teacher, social worker, or any similar person.

Local child protection procedures are clear [4], stating that all referrals of concern should be initially made to the social services department. Once inquiries have been made and it is agreed that an investigation should be entered into, the social workers concerned (who may be working in partnership with the police) should try to establish whether a child has suffered significant harm, or is at risk.

Usually, the parents will co-operate with the investigation and if the abuse has taken place, its nature will be assessable by the relevant professionals without recourse to legal action. It may be that, on occasions, parents will not allow the child to be assessed and are not amenable to persuasion or reasoning. If this refusal coincides with concerns that the child's health and welfare will be significantly harmed by a failure to establish if, and what, abuse is taking place, consideration should be given to applying for the child assessment order.

The court will have to be satisfied that the local authority has endeavoured to investigate the child's circumstances as fully as possible and this will include liaison with all the professional agencies involved with the child, in particular health professionals. All individuals who have knowledge of the child and his family should be included in the investigation and their opinion sought. Health visitors and general practitioners, for example, often have in-depth, ongoing knowledge of children and their families and are able to offer invaluable information to the investigation team.

Parents may feel more able to trust the family doctor or health visitor and on discussion with them agree to an assessment being completed. Equally, information may be available to the health professionals which clarifies particular queries or areas of doubt which the investigators may have. While skilled, experienced, social workers may be able to make sound assessments as to the child's emotional state and social conditions, including obvious changes in the child's physical well-being, they are not likely to have the specialist knowledge which may be needed to assess the complex areas surrounding particular physical or psychological symptoms. Such information is often vital, particularly in assessments of very young children who may be failing to thrive or where there are suspicions of sexual abuse.

STEPS TOWARDS APPLICATION

Once the investigation is under way and it appears that the parents are not willing to co-operate with the assessment, social services should convene a conference under the child protection procedures in order to review the progress of the investigation. Where the child has been assessed and the parents have co-operated, this conference can properly form a view about any potential level of risk. If the parents do not permit an assessment, the conference should consider how best to proceed. All relevant parties should be involved and pool what information they have. The role of the family doctor and health visitor should never be underestimated in these situations. Their knowledge of children and families is often based on contact that goes back prior to the birth of a particular child, and information they have very often clarifies many areas of concern for other professionals.

It can be concluded that if a child's best interests are to be served, positive relationships should exist between all parties involved with the child and that no individual party should under- (or over-) estimate the importance of his or her own contribution, or that of the other parties. All too often, inquiries into child-deaths or reports into incidents such as the Cleveland [5] and Rochdale [6] affairs, highlight breakdowns in the relationships not just between parents and professional agencies but between professionals themselves. Therefore, if an expectation exists that a child needs a particular specialist assessment, the relevant specialists should be involved from the earliest possible stages. This should include consultation as to how best the assessment should proceed in order to establish what is happening to the child, and where possible engaging the parents in the process. Practitioners should always try to attend child protection conferences and reviews when invited.

RECORDING THE PROCESS

The social services department, as lead agency in the investigation, has prime responsibility for recording all the steps which have been taken with both parents and with professional colleagues, but this should not undermine the importance of others recording their actions, involvement, or professional views as soon as possible. Child protection practice is complex and stressful, and perceptions of events are subject to personal interpretation and change. Memory can become clouded, opinions may alter or differ from those of others, or particular events suddenly gain a new significance. A written note is an invaluable guide as to how the attempts to assess the child have progressed.

WHO DOES THE ASSESSMENT?

The child protection conference, having established that an assessment is in the best interests of the child and that the parents are not co-operating, may then recommend further action. Given that this may lead to an application to the court for a child assessment order, it should be agreed as to who exactly will carry out the assessment. It may be that particular specialists such as paediatricians or psychiatrists are required. If this is likely to be the case, they should be included prior to and during the child protection conference so that their views are ascertained throughout and they can confirm their future availability.

It is the responsibility of the local authority in applying for this order to plan arrangements in advance so that the court can be satisfied that time-limits will be met and the appropriate professionals will be available. Such planning is not designed to present the court with a *fait accompli*, but to ensure that once intervention is authorised, delays are kept to a minimum.

The court will have to take advice as to how the assessment is to proceed. A guardian ad litem will be appointed to represent the best interests of the child and to advise. An assessment can be multi-disciplinary, including the child's emotional, medical, social, educational, and behavioural status; or more specific, such as psychiatric or a nutritional view of the child's needs, or a thorough examination by the family doctor.

ROLE OF THE GUARDIAN AD LITEM

The guardian ad litem will want to be satisfied on a number of points before advising the court. These will include the necessity for the assessment (which may mean discussions with the various specialists involved), meeting with the parents to establish that they fully understand what is expected but still disagree, and establishing for themselves whether they believe an assessment is in the child's best interests. They will have to take into account the age and abilities of the child to ascertain whether he has sufficient understanding to make an informed decision as to refusal or consent to the examination. If the child does have sufficient understanding and refuses to consent, the guardian must report this to the court. Such a judgment may be complex, particularly if there is a communication difficulty, and the guardian may wish to seek expert specialist advice in such cases.

Parents may request that their own practitioner be present during an examination of the child and the court may consent. This is aimed at preventing children having to undergo several examinations when one should be sufficient to ascertain their needs.

DIRECTIONS OF THE COURT

If the court is fully satisfied that the child is in need of assessment and that the parents remain uncooperative, an order will be made. The directions of the court will include such detail as the kind of assessment and the reason for it; who is to do the assessment and where; who will accompany the child, and who may specify the persons to whom the results should be given. Occasionally, it may be felt that a child should remain away from home during the assessment. If such an occasion arises, the court must ensure that this is not being used as an alternative to an emergency protection order.

A number of criteria are required for agreement to one or more overnight stays away from home of a child for observation purposes. As well as the court being satisfied as to its necessity, any periods away from home should be within the time-limits of the order. Proper contact between the child and his parents will have to be maintained and it may be believed that it is in the child's best interests that his parents stay with him overnight. Other parties may also need to have contact. The guardian will be expected to advise the court on this. Circumstances where overnight observations are vital may include those when the eating, sleeping, or other particular behaviour of the child need to be observed. Those who consider a stay away from home necessary will have to be very clear in their reasons why.

THE TIMING OF THE ASSESSMENT

The court can allow up to seven days for the assessment and the order will include the date from which it is to commence. Details of timing and all the relevant arrangements will have to be provided so that the court can be satisfied that the child's best interests are being met and that the assessment will be carried out within the time-limits. If, during the assessment, it is believed that the child is suffering such significant harm that he should not return home, an emergency protection order will have to be applied for. Equally, it may be that the court is so concerned about the child during the hearing, that it makes an emergency protection order instead of granting a child assessment order. This decision may be reached after hearing all the evidence and consequently reaching the view that the child's best interests are not met by that child remaining at home in the short term. The recommendation of the guardian will carry weight in the court.

Because of the time-limits, it is likely that the main emphasis of an initial assessment will be medical or psychiatric whereas, ideally, the order should at least include medical and social assessments; social assessments often taking longer to formulate. Medical assessments are often informed by social factors, but where a full social assessment is impossible, any specific social issues should be addressed in order to facilitate health work. This will include the race, culture, religion and gender of the child and his parents, information about housing status, any known family history, including disabilities, finances, education, or any other relevant information.

RACE AND CULTURE

All parties need to be aware of the idiosyncrasies of race, religion, culture and gender and the plans for any assessment should take these matters into account. The guardian will want to be assured that these factors have been fully addressed throughout the process, including the initial contacts with the child and family. It may be, for example, that the advice of health professionals from a particular racial or cultural group should be sought to clarify any assumptions that may, or may not, be made about attitudes towards physical examination. Language difficulties must be addressed and where English is not the first language, every effort should be made to ensure that the parents and child understand fully what is being asked of them, why, and the possible outcomes of particular courses of action. This applies equally where there may be communication difficulties with the child or parent for organic or other reasons.

FAILURE TO PRODUCE THE CHILD

Given that parents may understand fully the implications of refusing to allow an assessment to take place, they may fail to produce the child following the granting of a child assessment order. If this happens, an emergency protection order, interim care order or an interim supervision order with conditions may be sought. If the child refuses to submit to an assessment examination, either medical or psychiatric, and is of sufficient understanding, the court is not expected to try and change the child's mind and no party should pressurise the child.

CONCLUSION

All the above requirements indicate that a particular pattern of practice is expected when applying for child assessment orders. That is: constant referral to the child and his parents; co-operation between the professionals; clear planning at all stages; working with the guardian ad litem to establish what is in the best interests of the child; using the court only when not to do so would be harmful to the child; endeavouring to assess if the child is suffering from significant harm; taking into account the child's and parents' race, culture, religion, gender and any disabilities.

REFERENCES

1. Children Act 1989, s 47(3)(b)
2. Ibid, s 43
3. *A Child in Mind – Report into the Death of Kimberley Carlile* (London Borough of Greenwich, 1987)
4. See local Area Child Protection Committee, Inter-Agency Child Protection Procedures
5. *Report of the Inquiry into Child Abuse in Cleveland* (Cmnd 12, 1988)
6. Social Services Inspectorate *Report on Child Protection Practice in Rochdale* (HMSO, 1991)

Chapter 9

PROVISION OF RESOURCES FOR CHILDREN IN NEED

INTRODUCTION

Part III of the Act concerns the provision of services for children with disabilities and for children in need. It emphasises the role of families in caring for their children with, when necessary, the support of the local authority, by the provision of a range of services appropriate to the child's needs [1].

Local authorities have vested in them a general duty to safeguard and promote the welfare of children in their area who are in need. So far as is consistent with that duty, the local authority should promote the up-bringing of those children within their own families.

DEFINITIONS OF NEED

The Act sub-divides need into three categories: (1) the child is unlikely to achieve or maintain, or have the opportunity to achieve or maintain, a reasonable standard of health or development without the provision of services; (2) the child is likely to suffer significant impairment of his health or development without the provision of services; or (3) the child is disabled.

'Health' includes physical or mental health whereas 'development' could be physical, intellectual, emotional, social or behavioural development.

The definition of family is broader than the concept of parent–child. It includes any person who has parental responsibility for the child [2] and any other person with whom the child has been living. 'Family' can therefore include people who are not necessarily relatives.

Disability is defined as blindness, deafness, dumbness, or suffering from a mental disorder of any kind, or if the child is 'substantially and permanently handicapped by illness, injury or congenital deformity or such other disability as may be prescribed' [3]. It should be noted that this definition of disability, regrettably, does not include temporary medical conditions.

The importance of these definitions is that they not only reflect those definitions which are used for adults [4] but also that local authorities must include both those children who are neglected and those children with disabilities in the realm of their responsibilities. Within the terms of the Act, local authorities must not discriminate between the two when defining need.

DISCRETIONARY AND NON-DISCRETIONARY POWERS AND DUTIES

Local authorities have a number of duties placed upon them in relation to children in need. Whereas some of these are qualified duties, there are also some unqualified duties; practitioners should be aware of the local authorities' statutory responsibilities and their provision of services.

Two absolute duties are established. First, the local authority must open and maintain a register of children with disabilities within its area (parents have a final right of decision as to whether their child should be included on the register). Secondly, local authorities must provide published information as to the existence of appropriate services provided within their area. Further duties are established but are qualified, ie not compulsory.

THE REGISTER OF DISABLED CHILDREN

A number of factors have to be taken into account when compiling such a register. Clearly, decisions have to be made as to which children's names are to be entered on it. Once a child is considered disabled, both the parents and the child, if of sufficient understanding, have a right of veto over inclusion [5].

Local authorities' registers, in the past, have not always shown themselves to have been of benefit to those whose names are on them. Registration under the Chronically Sick and Disabled Persons Act 1970 does not appear to have guaranteed provision of services, nor does the maintenance of a register seem to have been proactive. Often, registration takes place as a reaction to service need. Child protection registers do not necessarily have a public image of value, and some children whose names are on them continue to be abused or neglected. Parents of children on this register often view their child's inclusion as negative and a means by which the child can be more easily removed from their care.

If a register of disability exists, logically it is expected that inclusion on it will facilitate the provision of appropriate resources.

Any register concerning children with disabilities should, ideally, be coordinated between the various agencies providing such services. This includes the local education and health authorities and the social services department. The register would then command an integrated assessment, rather than a number of separate non-coordinated assessments of the child's needs. This would underline all agencies' responsibilities to further the best interests of the child. It would also, it is hoped, create a register which was seen to be of value to the child and family and which was not critical of the parent's ability to care for the child.

Although it is ultimately the responsibility of the local authority to compile and maintain such a register, individual practitioners should advise families who are not aware of its existence. In the spirit of partnership and best practice the practitioner can offer information and advice to the family vis-à-vis referral, assessment and the reason for registration. Practitioners have a responsibility under the Act to promote the best interests of the child and inclusion on the register should facilitate this.

INFORMATION ABOUT SERVICES

The local authority, having a duty to provide information about services for children in need, should have due regard to ensuring the proper distribution and comprehensibility of that information. Practitioners should endeavour to obtain the information and when they believe that the family cannot understand it for any reason, they should inform the local authority. Translated versions may be needed for example, and the provision of Braille or taped copies encouraged.

THE CHILD AND THE FAMILY

Local authorities have a general duty to promote the upbringing of children by their families. Services should be supportive of families rather than a substitute for care within them.

Services can range from practical support, such as a home help, to the provision of information and advice to families. Basically, whatever steps might be thought appropriate should be considered. The advice of practitioners might be sought in order to assess the appropriateness of resources, or they may wish to advise local authorities as to their views about the resource needs of a particular child.

When a child is not living with his family and is being looked after by the local authority, the local authority has a duty to facilitate that child's return to his family or to establish appropriate contact with the family. This has to be assessed in the light of safeguarding or promoting the child's welfare.

ACCOMMODATION OF CHILDREN BY THE LOCAL AUTHORITY

There may be occasions when the local authority and a child's parents agree that the child's best interests are not being served by his remaining in the family home at that time. The local authority then has a responsibility to consider offering to accommodate that child.

Accommodation is seen as a supportive mechanism to maintain the child in need within the family in the longer term. When children are accommodated, the local authority, working in partnership with the parents, does not acquire parental responsibility. Accommodation should usually be seen as a short-term resolution to a particular difficulty, fully involving those with parental responsibility in decisions about the child. The new philosophy of accommodation negates previous requirements of 28 days' notice being given by a parent wishing to discharge a child from a voluntary arrangement.

When a child is to be accommodated, it is expected that written agreements are entered into between the parents and the local authority. Agreements should contain details concerning the resources to be provided by the local authority; contact with the parents; appropriate education; proposed duration of accommodation; relationships with other agencies; and any other relevant factors. Agreements, although not legally binding in themselves, could, of course, be used as evidence in legal proceedings and need to be treated with proper seriousness by all parties.

THE PROVISION OF FAMILY CENTRES

In order to prevent the need for a child to be accommodated, care proceedings being initiated, or, most importantly, to provide relevant resources for children in need, local authorities have a duty to provide such family centres as they feel appropriate. These are centres where a family may attend for occupational, social, cultural or recreational activities; for advice, guidance or counselling; or be provided with accommodation while receiving these services. These centres can have residential provision.

Many local authorities already provide family centres either directly or in partnership with voluntary agencies. Practitioners may advise the local authority as to how family centres can be designed to best protect the interests of children in need in their area. Practitioners may be included in the teams offering services from such centres.

It is important to note that this is the first time that family centres have been so described in legislation and this is an indication of the Act's philosophy which encourages the maintenance of children within their families. When plans are being made, therefore, the use of family centres should be properly considered.

THE PROVISION OF DAY CARE

Local authorities are also required to provide day care, as is appropriate, for children in need who are under the age of five and not yet attending school. It can also be provided for children who are not considered to be in need. It does not have to be on a regular basis, being defined more as supervised activity or care provided for children during the day.

As the local authority can define provision in terms of appropriateness, practitioners should not only be aware of what day care is available but should also be advising the local authority as to appropriate ways of meeting the needs of children locally.

THE PREVENTION OF ABUSE AND NEGLECT

The general duties of local authorities to safeguard and promote the welfare of children, and their more specific responsibilities outlined in Part III of the Act (both in terms of maintaining, where possible, children in their families, and providing resources for children in need), accords with the spirit of the legislation at a variety of levels. These duties acknowledge that the prevention of abuse and neglect is not something which should be automatically associated with recourse to the courts. Court action should only be resorted to when the child's interests are being adversely affected by any significant harm which the child may be suffering, or is likely to suffer.

These principles can lead to the realisation that the provision of particular resources, in conjunction with an atmosphere of partnership between parents and the agencies concerned, can proactively address potential abuse and neglect. When necessary, resources should be available to meet the needs of children who have been abused or neglected; wherever possible, abuse or neglect should be prevented in the first place. Access to appropriate resources may further this aim.

If practitioners are of the view that a child is not maintaining, or is not likely to maintain a reasonable standard of health or development, they should refer to the local authority as early as possible in the process of their assessment; this should, of course, be in negotiation with the parents. This is more likely to ensure the provision of appropriate resources, as planning for the child's needs can take place and timely provision be considered. Consequently, the child should be less likely to suffer due to the various agencies' inability to perceive and provide resources at the right time. It is also potentially more conducive to positive parent–agency relationships if open communication prevails. Generally, parents do not abuse or neglect children out of vindictiveness or carelessness. The family, or parent, is often under stress for a variety of reasons which may be financial, environmental, social, medical, psychological, or a mixture of factors. These, in themselves, may lead to an assessment that a child is in need and in addressing this the agencies must properly confront the prevailing circumstances. Parents are then in a position to see that it is the needs of their child which are being considered, and not that they are on trial.

RACE AND CULTURE

Local authorities should take full and proper regard of a child's race and culture when making provision for day care [6], and more generally should do so when developing strategies to implement any policies regarding the welfare of children.

There are many areas of need in which racial and cultural factors should properly be considered. For example, although many disabilities or medical conditions are experienced by all children, whatever their racial origin, some are more prevalent in particular racial groups. When this is the case and members of those groups live in a particular area, all agencies should consider how best they can advise and support those families which may be affected.

When accommodating a child the local authority must give proper regard to that child's racial and cultural background when seeking placement. An understanding of the support that is available to families in their communities and an assessment as to whether they are appropriate in particular cases may avoid the need for accommodation. For example, this may include extended families whose members, such as grandparents, can be very helpful in the provision of child care, as can relevant community-based groups.

Conversely, when families are separated from their cultural groups, they may experience stress and potential breakdown of the family due to the absence of extended family members or community support. Practitioners in areas where there are new housing developments or regular changes of population should be aware of this.

Where there are language differences, interpreters should be available so that adequate assessments of need can take place. A parent may not be able, due to language difficulties for example, to describe in detail a child's symptomology or responses to various stimulations. Practitioners may, therefore, feel less able to give an assured opinion, or decide that more extensive assessments are needed.

Different cultures have different patterns of relationships between lay people and the 'authorities', the sexes, other racial groups, and any variety of social and interpersonal settings. Not all professionals can be aware of all cultural differences, but each has a responsibility, when possible, to inform others of any differences. They also need to understand that behaviour may be influenced by such patterns of relationships rather than by negative attitudes. Further to this, understatements concerning the severity of symptoms or behavioural patterns may be being made.

THE ROLE OF THE MEDICAL PRACTITIONER

Practitioners are an integral part of a team assessing needs of children, both individually and within groups. Clearly, it may be that the most easily defined group of children in need are those with disabilities. A variety of assessment systems already exist and social services departments, and education and health authorities where possible, may elect to operate integrated systems of assessment and registration.

Practitioners have a role in advising all relevant agencies how best they can tailor particular services to ensure provision for children in need.

On an individual basis, a child, although not having a disability, may be assessed as being in need and a medical opinion will often be sought. Practitioners should understand that it is as necessary to establish that a child is healthy as it is that he is unhealthy. On occasions, practitioners may have to remind colleagues from other disciplines of this. General practitioners and members of primary health teams will often have knowledge of the medical history of a child and family over a long period of time and in depth. This, combined with social, psychological and behavioural assessments, will greatly enhance evaluations of need.

STATUTORY DUTY TO CO-OPERATE

The Act [7] empowers the local authority to request help, from health authorities among others, in the exercise of any of its functions defined in Part III. Necessary action has to be identified and specifically requested, preferably in writing. The health authority should comply unless it is incompatible with its own statutory and other duties or prejudices the discharge of any of its other functions.

VOLUNTARY AGENCIES

The local authority may make any arrangements that it sees fit, with any person, to act on its behalf in the provision of services for children in need. This may be other statutory authorities or the voluntary sector.

Many voluntary organisations exist to offer specialist services to children in need, including children with disabilities. The ethos of the Act is such that the local authority is positively encouraged to establish relationships with these organisations, particularly when their role facilitates the continued care of children in their families.

CONCLUSION

Part III of the Act sets out those services which the local authorities must, or may, provide for children or their families. Most importantly, it brings together the services which may be provided for children in need and for children with disabilities, recognising that disability is in itself sufficient to establish need.

The emphasis is on children remaining, where possible, within their families, with support when necessary. If this is not possible, families may negotiate with the local authority for their child to be looked after in accommodation. Usually, this is with a view to the child returning home as soon as is possible.

Practitioners will often be fully involved in assessments of need, whether or not the child has a disability. They may advocate on behalf of the child or family for the provision of particular services by the local authority or its appointees.

Due consideration should be given to the racial and cultural needs of children, both when assessments take place and in provision of services and general family support.

All practitioners are positively encouraged to work together in partnership, both with each other and the families concerned.

REFERENCES

1. Children Act 1989, s 17
2. See Chapter 2
3. Children Act 1989, s 17(11)
4. National Assistance Act 1948, s 29(1)
5. See White, Carr and Lowe *A Guide to The Children Act 1989* (supplement to *Clarke Hall & Morrison on Children)* (Butterworths, 1990) p 59
6. Children Act 1989, Sch 2, para 11
7. Ibid, s 27

Chapter 10

CONSENT TO MEDICAL EXAMINATIONS AND ASSESSMENT

Practitioners need to make a clear distinction between medical examination and treatment which is necessary for the health and welfare of a person, and examinations or assessments which are for forensic purposes, ie to produce evidence for a court. This chapter looks at both, in the light of the new legislation.

CONSENTS FOR MEDICAL EXAMINATION AND TREATMENT GENERALLY

Adults

No adult person may be given medical treatment without that person's consent. To do so, whatever the motive, may constitute an assault for which the practitioner may incur liability for damages in the law of tort, or may even constitute an offence in criminal law. Detention in hospital or any other place without consent could constitute false imprisonment, also giving rise to an action for damages in tort. There are, of course, exceptions.

In emergencies, where a person is incapable of giving or withholding consent (perhaps because he or she is unconscious) the doctor may proceed in treating the patient.

In two recent cases [1], judges have given guidance on in-patient treatment and specific medical interventions in the case of adults. The basis of the guidance is that where a patient is incapable of understanding the implications of treatment, or perhaps lacks insight into the nature and extent of their illness, out-patient treatment or medication should not be administered on a compulsory basis unless with the prior sanction of a

High Court judge. As Elizabeth Lawson QC pointed out [2], the liberty of the individual requires that treatment is only given compulsorily where a patient is so mentally ill or disordered that compulsory admission for hospital treatment is necessary in their best interests, under the Mental Health Act 1983, s 3.

Detention for in-patient treatment of mental illness and compulsory administration of medication or other surgical treatment is regulated by further statutory safeguards in the Mental Health Act 1983, ss 57 and 58.

Re F [1] involved the issue of compulsory sterilisation for an adult with the mental capacity of a young child who was argued to be incapable of understanding pregnancy or child-rearing. It was stated that sterilisation would be in the patient's best interests. The court ducked the issue of directly dealing with consent by ruling that if the operation were to be performed, it would not be unlawful, thus giving the doctors involved, in a roundabout way, an immunity from consequential legal action against them for assault in criminal or civil law.

The recent case of Re GF [3] demonstrated that no application to the court is necessary for a declaration as to the lawfulness of a proposed therapeutic operation which would have the incidental effect of sterilisation of a woman incapable of consent, where the operation is necessary to improve or ensure the health of the patient. Two practitioners should be satisfied that:

(a) the operation is necessary for therapeutic purposes;
(b) it is in the best interests of the patient; and
(c) there is no practicable less intrusive means of treatment.

At what Age can a Person give Consent?

The question arises as to when a child becomes old enough to give his own consent: first, for medical, surgical or psychiatric treatment, and secondly, for an examination or assessment.

Childhood may be described as 'a state of steadily increasing ability' particularly in relation to medical decision-making. At the age of 16 [4], a young person gains the absolute right to give informed consent to surgical, medical or dental treatment. Examinations or assessments could also impliedly be included.

A young person aged 16 or over who has a mental illness, disability, or psychiatric disturbance will be subject to the same mental health provisions and safeguards as an adult.

However, although the right to consent to medical treatment is clear, the right to refuse treatment which has been advised by doctors is less clear. Two recent cases illustrate the difficulty for both practitioners and the courts.

In *Re J* [1992] *The Times*, 15 May, a local authority having the care of J, a 16-year-old girl suffering from anorexia, applied to the High Court under the Act for an order within the High Court's inherent jurisdiction granting leave to treat her compulsorily, following the girl's refusal to accept the medical treatment recommended to her. It was submitted to the court that J was of sufficient understanding to make her own decision. It was also argued that since a child may make an informed refusal of examinations and assessments under certain provisions of the Act, if the spirit of the Act is followed in general practice, a child should also be able to refuse treatment provided that she is able to make an informed decision. The judge in this case followed the earlier decision in the case of *Re R* [4], that consent could be taken from any of those persons entitled to give it, and that the High Court has power to overrule a minor even if she is '*Gillick* competent' [5]. Therefore, the judge ordered that treatment be given.

From the information available at the time of writing, it seems that the arguments in *Re J* (above) were based mainly on analogy with the provisions of the Act relating to examination and assessment in child protection cases.

These situations could perhaps be approached in a different way. If a person suffers from anorexia and this condition were to continue untreated, that person would almost certainly suffer considerable general discomfort and possibly also long-term damage to vital organs. A severe untreated case may even result in death. In these circumstances, expert evidence could be called to assess the patient's current mental state, also giving any available background information about the relevant psychological factors leading to the onset of the condition. The court could then consider whether this person is suffering from a mental illness of a type which would justify compulsory treatment under the Mental Health Acts. If compulsory treatment proved unjustified on this basis, the court would then have to choose between alternative approaches.

The first, 'non-interventionist' approach is that if the young patient were then adjudged to be '*Gillick* competent' (ie under 16 and capable of making an informed decision), or over 16 years of age, she should be able to make her own decision as to her treatment, in the same way as any similarly competent adult. The Family Law Reform Act 1969, s 8(1), after all, enables a person over 16 to give valid legal consent to treatment. Theoretically, this concept could also be extended to allow a '*Gillick* competent' child's refusal to be respected.

The second, perhaps more paternalistic alternative, is to utilise the inherent jurisdiction of the High Court to override the will of any person under 18 where it is deemed necessary for their health and welfare. At present, the courts seem to be prepared to take this course with a person under 18, and in a recent case, also with an adult.

In *Re T*, a 20-year-old woman was admitted to hospital following an accident. She had, before losing consciousness, expressed a clear refusal of blood transfusions on religious grounds. Her family was divided on the issue. The Court of Appeal, in July 1992, confirmed a decision of the High Court to authorise treatment for her by blood transfusion. In considering medical treatment, the courts, so far, have respected the clearly expressed wish of an adult who is fully in possession of his reasoning ability, ie in legal terms, 'compos mentis'. When full reports of this case are available, it will be interesting to study the full facts and reasons for this decision.

In *Re J (A Minor) (Medical Treatment)* [1992] 2 FLR 165, the Court of Appeal, in June 1992, reaffirmed the principle that in the exercise of its inherent power to protect the interests of minors it will not compel a medical practitioner or a health authority to adopt a course of treatment which, in the bona fide clinical judgment of the practitioner, is contra-indicated as not being in the patient's best interests. In this case, Lord Donaldson MR said that it would be an abuse of power for a court directly or indirectly to require a doctor to act contrary to his professional duty. That duty is, subject to necessary consent, to treat the patient in accordance with his own best clinical judgment, notwithstanding that other practitioners not called to treat the patient, or the court, acting on expert evidence, might disagree. Here, a paediatrician caring for a profoundly mentally and physically handicapped baby with a short life expectancy, advised that intervention with artificial ventilation procedures would not be appropriate if the baby suffered a life-threatening event. The court refused to order such treatment.

Children under the Age of 16

Gillick Competence: When can a Child under the Age of 16 give Consent?

The 'increasing ability' of childhood has been formally recognised by the courts in a number of recent cases, the most famous of which was the *Gillick* case [5]. Mrs Gillick requested her local area health authority not to give contraceptive advice or treatment to her daughters while they were still under the age of 16 without her express consent. The health authority preferred to place full reliance upon the doctor's medical judgment in each individual case, and refused to act otherwise. Mrs Gillick sought through the courts to declare this refusal unlawful. The case went to the House of Lords because it involved a point of law of public importance. The Law Lords had to decide whether a child under the age of 16 could give a valid consent for medical examination and treatment. In giving judgment, they formulated the basis of the concept now known colloquially as '*Gillick* competence' in which the ability of a child under the age of 16 to make his own medical decisions is evaluated according to chronological age, considered in conjunction with the child's mental and emotional maturity, intelligence and comprehension. Clearly, this will not steadily increase with chronological age, but will variably increase according to the individual. The graph below (Figure 10.1) indicates the general pattern, but not the individual detail, of the increase of '*Gillick* competence'.

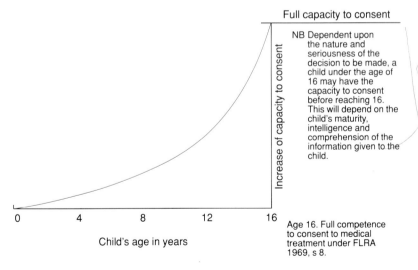

Full capacity to consent

NB Dependent upon the nature and seriousness of the decision to be made, a child under the age of 16 may have the capacity to consent before reaching 16. This will depend on the child's maturity, intelligence and comprehension of the information given to the child.

Increase of capacity to consent

0   4   8   12   16

Child's age in years

Age 16. Full competence to consent to medical treatment under FLRA 1969, s 8.

Variables: intelligence, understanding, information given

Figure 10.1   Illustration of the concept of Gillick competence

The principles of the *Gillick* case were reviewed in a number of subsequent cases, including *Re E* and *Re R* [6]. In *Re E*, a 15-year-old boy refused on religious grounds to allow for himself a life-saving blood transfusion, but the court overrode his refusal on the grounds that he had not yet reached sufficient understanding to make the decision. In *Re R*, the child was a girl of 15 years and 10 months. She had been known to social services for a long time, and was known to have periodic mental disturbance and psychotic episodes. Her history was one of being at risk, and it was suspected that she had suffered from emotional abuse. The question for the High Court was whether she should be given medication for her mental state when she did not wish to take it. The court decided (despite evidence from her psychiatrist to the contrary) that she could not give an informed refusal, and that decision was subsequently upheld on appeal.

These cases have generated much comment and thought by those who have to seek or comply with consents for medical, surgical, psychiatric or other treatments.

Lord Scarman felt that the decision was one of fact in each case. He said in the *Gillick* case:

'It will be a question of fact whether a child seeking advice has sufficient understanding of what is involved to give a consent valid in law. Until the child achieves the capacity to consent, the parental right to make the decision continues save only in exceptional circumstances. Emergency, parental neglect, abandonment of the child, or inability to find the parent are examples of exceptional situations.'

Clearly, the relative importance of the decision to be made will affect the child's capacity to consent. Very young children find it difficult to see themselves and their own situation in a wider social and physical context, and they also find it hard to conceptualise. The ability to understand and assess the potential consequences of having (or refusing) treatment or assessment will usually increase with age and maturity, although it will, of course, be affected by other factors such as the information provided for the child upon which to base the decision, the child's intelligence and level of understanding.

The ability to make a valid legal decision about a dental examination may be reached at an earlier chronological age than a decision about major surgery.

It will usually be the doctor who provides the information for the patient, and who also assesses the ability of a child to make a valid decision. The NHS guidelines [7] are that the doctor should record carefully the factors taken into account by the doctor in making his assessment of the child's capacity to give a valid consent. It is strongly recommended that doctors go further than these recommendations and also record carefully the substance of the factual information given to the child, including the questions asked and the child's responses. A record such as this would be invaluable not only for the medical notes but also for possible reference later if the child's ability to make the decision were to be questioned.

The NHS guidance [8] recommends that where a child is seen alone, efforts should be made to persuade the child that his parents should be informed, except in circumstances where it is clearly not in the child's best interests. It reiterates the need for parental consent in cases where a child under the age of 16 cannot make a valid decision for himself, except in an emergency.

Practitioners should be aware of the rights and duties of those with parental responsibility for children. Unfortunately, no reference is made to this in the current edition of the NHS guidance.

Mentally Ill or Mentally Disordered Children

Where a child is mentally ill or mentally disordered, and is unable to understand the implications of the suggested treatment, that child may not be able to make a legally valid decision for himself. The High Court has, in its wardship jurisdiction, the power to consent on behalf of a person under the age of 18, and has done so in recent decided cases such as Re B [9]. In this case, the court consented to the sterilisation of a young woman with learning disabilities. The case was similar to that of Re F described above, but here, even though the girl was over 16 years old, the court held that it had power to give consent in her best interests, because she was mentally incapable of making her own decision.

There are safeguards in the Mental Health Act 1983 for the mentally disordered child as there are for adults. Parents can arrange [10] for the informal admission of children under the age of 16 to hospital for treatment for mental disorder, and for the admission for those over the age of 16 if they are incapable of making their own decisions or expressing their own wishes.

The definition of 'nearest relative' in the Mental Health Act 1983 [11] is now amended to substitute for the word 'mother' both mother and father who have parental responsibility for the child within the meaning of s 3 of the Children Act 1989.

Parental Responsibility and Consent

The Act changes the status of parents in relation to their children, and that of children themselves concerning many matters. Decision-making powers no longer rest with parents simply by virtue of their having given birth to a child. They need to have parental responsibility for that child in order to make legal decisions in respect of that child. The Act, however, makes a special provision for those who have the care of a child but do not have parental responsibility:

'A person who –

(a) does not have parental responsibility for a particular child; but
(b) has care of the child,

may . . . do what is reasonable in all the circumstances of the case for the purpose of safeguarding or promoting the child's welfare.' [12]

The definition of parental responsibility, its effects, and the ways in which it may be acquired or lost, are discussed in Chapter 2.

Parental Responsibility, Medical Records and Consent Issues

It will be evident that medical records should now take into account information as to who has parental responsibility for each child. A significant percentage of children are born into families where their parents are unmarried, and in these cases it is quite possible that only the mother will have parental responsibility for the child. The child's father may have acquired it, and if so, should be able to produce a stamped copy of the parental responsibility agreement, or a copy of a court order, to demonstrate his status in relation to his child, which can then be noted in the child's medical records.

In circumstances where a father brings a child for examination or treatment to the general practitioners or to the hospital, and it is not an emergency, his ability to give, legally, the appropriate consents for treatment may need to be checked against the records held at the surgery or hospital. This also applies to a non-parent. Clearly, the special provision in s 3(5) cited above may provide the power for a parent or non-parent without parental responsibility to consent to treatment for a child, but practitioners should be cautious about its use where treatment is not urgent.

For children living away from home, whether with relatives or in local authority accommodation, situations may arise where consents are required and where the issue of parental responsibility in the child's records may prove to be important.

PROBLEM SITUATIONS

What if a *'Gillick* Competent' Child Decides, but Parent(s) Disagree?

1. One or Both Parents Refuse, but Child Consents

In the case of *Re R* in 1991, [13], the Court of Appeal referred to the *Gillick* case, and considered the position of a child who, although under the age of 16, was competent to make legally valid decisions, but whose parent(s) differed in their views from those of the child. Lord Donaldson indicated that the child, if *'Gillick* competent', acquires a right to make decisions equal to that of each of his parents. His view expressed in *Re R* was that there can be concurrent powers to consent, and that only a failure to, or refusal of, consent by all of those having that power would create a veto.

It was also said in *Re R* that no doctor can be required to treat a child, whether by consent of the court in the exercise of its wardship jurisdiction, or by the consent of the parents or the child or anyone else. The decision whether to treat a child is dependent upon the exercise of the doctor's own professional judgment, subject only to the threshold requirement that, save in exceptional cases, usually an emergency, the doctor has the consent of someone who has the authority to give it. In forming this judgment, the views and wishes of the child are factors which have increasing importance in accordance with the increase in the child's intelligence and understanding.

The NHS guidance clearly recognises the principle that:

'Where a child under the age of sixteen achieves a sufficient understanding of what is proposed, the child may consent to a doctor or health professional making an examination and giving treatment. The doctor or health professional must be satisfied that any such child has sufficient understanding of what is involved in the treatment which is proposed.' [14]

The factors taken into account in making the decision should also be carefully noted in the practitioner's records.

2. *One or Both Parents Consent, but Child Refuses*

At the time of writing it has been left open whether a '*Gillick* competent' child's refusal of treatment is absolute.

In *Re R*, Lord Donaldson seems to have implied that if such a child refuses treatment, the doctor could still lawfully proceed if the necessary consent were to be obtained from another legally competent source.

If the parents themselves differ in opinion, impliedly then, the doctor may take the permission of the one who agrees provided that the doctor considers that the treatment is necessary and in the best interests of the patient. This argument may seem viable where the child agrees to the treatment, but where a '*Gillick* competent' child refuses medical intervention, would it be right to force treatment upon that child, even if a parent wishes it? Irrespective of legal niceties, there is a moral and ethical dilemma. Could a doctor, having decided that a child is able to give an informed decision, then ignore that child's informed refusal? Many doctors take the view that the only viable way through such a dilemma is negotiation with the child and with the parents in the hope that a workable agreement will be reached. If this proves impossible, most doctors would not then proceed to examine or treat a child who gives an informed refusal unless their condition were dangerous or life threatening. The NHS guidance [14] clearly states that the refusal of an adult or competent young person must be respected.

The case of *Re R* took place before the implementation of the Children Act 1989 and, therefore, the comments made by the Court of Appeal must be modified by the provisions of the new legislation. 'Parents' would now have to be substituted by 'those who have parental responsibility for the child'; and there is now an added dimension because there are specific provisions in the Children Act relating to medical examination and assessments, discussed below.

Where practitioners encounter problems with medical treatment or examination of a child which cannot be resolved by negotiation, a specific issue order under s 8 of the Act may be sought. The legal department of the local authority for the area in which the child lives should be able to advise. The local authority, the child's parents, or anyone with leave of the court (including the child if of sufficient understanding), may apply for an order.

POWER OF THE HIGH COURT IN WARDSHIP OR ITS INHERENT JURISDICTION TO OVERRIDE DECISIONS OF PARENTS, CHILD OR OTHERS

Would the High Court Override a *'Gillick* Competent' Child's Refusal?

In theory, it is possible for the High Court in its wardship jurisdiction to override the wishes of anyone else in relation to the ward of court. This will include the possibility of overriding the wishes of the ward himself, *'Gillick* competent' or not. The court places the child's welfare of paramount importance, making its decision in the best interests of the ward. It is, in theory, possible for wardship to be used to gain consent for (or prohibition of) any treatment or medical procedure for any young person under the age of 18 within the court's jurisdiction if this is considered by the court to be in the ward's best interests.

The High Court has an inherent jurisdiction which can be used, quite apart from wardship, to make a variety of orders including those under the Children Act 1989. Where there is a difficulty in resolving a dilemma relating to medical treatment for a child, it is now also possible to seek its resolution by a specific issue order under s 8 of the Act. The case of *Re J*, discussed at p 65 above, would seem to indicate that the High Court is prepared to overrule a child's refusal where treatment is considered necessary for the child's health and welfare.

THE NEW LEGISLATION: SPECIFIC PROVISIONS OF THE CHILDREN ACT 1989 RELATING TO MEDICAL OR PSYCHIATRIC EXAMINATION AND ASSESSMENT

In many circumstances, child protection will necessitate medical or psychiatric examinations or assessments of a child. It has become clear from the Cleveland affair and related research that repeated medical examinations can, in themselves, be abusive to children and so the Act enables the court, in specified circumstances, to control and, if need be, give directions concerning examinations, setting appropriate limits. The power of the court is wide. Directions could include the place and time of an examination, the person(s) to be present, the person(s) to conduct the examination, and the person(s) or authorities to whom the results shall be given.

These directions may be given when the court makes an interim care or supervision order, an emergency protection order or a child assessment order. The child who has sufficient understanding has a right to make an informed decision to refuse such an examination or assessment.

The Child's Rights under the Children Act 1989 to make an Informed Refusal of Medical Examination or Assessment

The whole ethos of the Act is that children are people with rights and powers, and that they have the right to be heard and have their wishes and feelings taken into account. On this basis, it was felt that there should be a right of refusal by children to certain medical and psychiatric examinations, provided that the decision was an informed one made by a child of sufficient understanding.

Where the court has the power to control medical examinations, and the child has the right to refuse, the child's wishes and feelings must be ascertained at the earliest possible opportunity. The best person to do this is the guardian ad litem, who will be appointed at as early a stage as possible in the proceedings. The doctor also has a responsibility, unspecified in the Act itself but clearly laid down in the *Guidance and Regulations* [15], to check whether the child is capable of giving an informed decision and that the child consents, before proceeding. It is hoped that the court will have had the time to ascertain the child's wishes and feelings before giving directions, but where the case has been urgent, there may not have been time and then the doctor's duty to check is vital.

The questions and answers between the practitioner and the child about consent should be recorded in whatever form is convenient, but it is recommended that a contemporaneous written note is made of the substance of questions and answers, also recording any relevant action taken. Should there be any question at a later stage as to the basis upon which the doctor advises that the child is or is not capable of giving an informed decision, then the grounds for that advice are clear. The information given by the doctor to the child should also be recorded. A child cannot make an informed decision without having been given appropriate information enabling the child to consider the proposals, the available alternatives and the potential consequences.

If after there have been directions given by the court, but when the child is with the doctor, the child refuses the examination, and the doctor feels that this is an informed decision, then the doctor should not proceed but should refer the matter back to the court. Courts are not, however, in the business of cajoling or persuading children to give consent.

If there have been no directions given as to a medical examination, and the doctor is faced with an informed refusal, the doctor should not proceed at that stage with the examination but refer the matter, if possible, back to the court. The court may ask the guardian ad litem and the doctor to help by discussing the matter fully with the child, and if it is agreed that the child's decision is an informed one, then it is submitted that the court will have to abide by it.

There are no guidelines in the Act as to how the ability to make informed decisions is to be ascertained – presumably the principles in *Gillick* and other cases will apply, looking at the child's chronological age in relation to his intelligence, level of understanding and ability to conceptualise, together with the information supplied to the child on which to base the decision. The potential consequences of a refusal may lead to a lack of evidence upon which to prosecute a case of suspected abuse, or even the taking of protective proceedings in relation to the child. Those making an assessment of a child's ability to refuse, will need to remember that the child may have been subjected to pressure by others to keep the alleged abuse a secret, or even to deny it altogether. The questions asked to elicit the child's decision will need to take these issues, and many other possibilities into account. Doctors, guardians ad litem and other experts, could profitably share their expertise when advising the court [16].

Can the Court Overrule a Child's Informed Refusal under the Children Act 1989?

The High Court is the upper tier of 'the court' created by the Act, therefore it is governed by the Act in exercising its powers in relation to children.

As discussed above, it seems that only the High Court has the potential power to override a child's informed refusal of examination or assessment under the Act. Each case would have to be decided upon its individual merits, but subject to the restrictions in the Act on the uses of wardship and the High Court's inherent jurisdiction [17].

The potential use of a specific issue order to resolve a difference of opinion between a child and parent(s) or doctors has already been discussed earlier in this chapter in the context of treatment in general medical practice. Treatment, which may be vital to the child's health and welfare, must be clearly distinguished from an examination and assessment which could be purely for forensic purposes.

It remains to be seen whether the courts would now override a child's decision under the Children Act 1989 to refuse consent for examination or assessment. So far, there have been no cases on this point, so it is possible only to guess at the decision the High Court would make in a case referred to it where a child has given an informed refusal under the Act, even if the court did not consider objectively that decision to be in the best interests of the child. The spirit of the Act demands that the court accepts and respects a child's informed refusal. However, as many doctors have pointed out, whatever a court said about it, they would not be willing to forcibly carry out, for example, an internal examination of a teenage female victim of alleged sexual abuse if she did not agree to it.

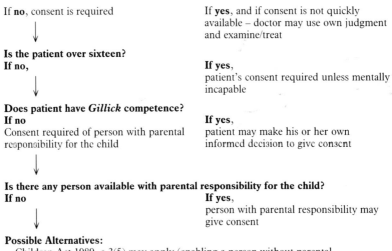

PRACTITIONER ADVISES MEDICAL TREATMENT
– IS THIS SITUATION AN EMERGENCY?

If **no**, consent is required

↓

Is the patient over sixteen?
If no,

↓

Does patient have *Gillick* competence?
If no
Consent required of person with parental
responsibility for the child

↓

If **yes**, and if consent is not quickly
available – doctor may use own judgment
and examine/treat

If yes,
patient's consent required unless mentally
incapable

If yes,
patient may make his or her own
informed decision to give consent

Is there any person available with parental responsibility for the child?
If no   **If yes,**
↓   person with parental responsibility may
                                       give consent

Possible Alternatives:
– Children Act 1989, s 3(5) may apply (enabling a person without parental responsibility to do what is necessary for the welfare of the child);
  or
– the court could appoint a guardian for a child who has no parent with parental responsibility for him;
  or
– the local authority may seek a court order under s 31 or emergency protection to give them parental responsibility for the child;
  or
– any relative or other person may seek a residence order and parental responsibility for the child, or any person may seek a specific issue order with leave of the court.

Figure 10.2 Consent Checklist for Necessary Medical Treatment

Note. This checklist relates only to medical treatment advised by the practitioner in the patient's interests and not to examination and assessments purely for forensic purposes.

REFERENCES

1. *R v Hallstrom and Another Ex Parte W* (1986) 2 All ER 306 and also *Re F* (1990) 2 AC 1
2. Article by Elizabeth Lawson QC 'Are Gillick Rights Under Threat?' in *Childright* October 1991, pp 17–21
3. *Re GF* [1991] FCR 776, sub nom *Re GF (Medical Treatment)* [1992] 1 FLR 293
4. Family Law Reform Act 1969, s 8
5. *Gillick v West Norfolk and Wisbech Area Health Authority and Another* (1986) AC 112, [1986] 1 FLR 224
6. *Re E (Wardship)* [1992] 2 FCR 219 and also *Re R (Wardship)*, CA [1992] 2 FCR 229, sub nom *Re R (A Minor) (Wardship: Medical Treatment)*, CA [1992] 1 FLR 190
7. *A Guide to Consent for Examination or Treatment* (NHS Management Executive)
8. Ibid, pp 4–5
9. *Re B (A Minor) (Wardship: Sterilisation)* (1988) AC 199
10. Mental Health Act 1983, s 131(2)
11. Mental Health Act 1983, s 27(2)
12. Children Act 1989, s 3(5)
13. *Re R (Wardship)*, CA [1992] 2 FCR 229, sub nom *Re R (A Minor) (Wardship: Medical Treatment)*, CA [1992] 1 FLR 190
14. *A Guide to Consent for Examination or Treatment* (NHS Management Executive) p 4
15. *Children Act 1989 Guidance and Regulations Volume 1 Court Orders* (HMSO, 1991)
16. *Working Together Under the Children Act* (HMSO, 1991)
17. Children Act 1989, s 100

Chapter 11

COMMUNICATING WITH CHILDREN AND ADOLESCENTS

INTRODUCTION

Many adults assume that they can communicate with children without difficulty. A number of those who do not make this assumption develop a variety of techniques in order to overcome the difficulty. These techniques vary from dominating the child, patronising the child, ignoring the child, or even behaving like the child.

The literal meaning of communication 'is to give to another as a partaker; to impart, confer, transmit'. None of these techniques achieves this. As 'partake' means to share, there is an assumption of reciprocity in the relationship, and it is the adult's responsibility to endeavour to ensure that any communication taking place is, where possible, on the child's terms; that is, child-centred, not childish.

The Act recognises this in various ways. Its first statement that the child's welfare is the paramount consideration lays the foundation for a child-centred approach. Its emphasis on consultation and partnership with families assumes that when agencies become involved, where possible they do so on the basis of negotiation.

AGE-APPROPRIATE LANGUAGE

The basis of a child-centred approach is to relate to children on a level which is appropriate to their age.

Practitioners will be aware that from birth, and before, children are affected by the environment around them. In relating to the child, the adult transmits non-verbal and verbal signals. The younger the child, the greater the need for the adult to give signals which create a positive relationship between adult and child and a general atmosphere of security. If the child does not feel secure, his reaction is likely to be alarm and the response to this is likely to be to cry despairingly. This in itself can make the adult more nervous and the child feel even less secure.

This may seem obvious, but it should be remembered that it is on the observation of the adult–child relationship that practitioners begin to assess how positively or negatively attached children are to their parents. It is through such observations that 'objective' opinions are reached.

In addition to the adult–child non-verbal relationship is the adult's use of language and voice modulation. Babyhood is an excellent reminder to adults about the relevance of tone of voice. Meaning is conveyed by the tone of the voice and the volume it is pitched at, as well as the specific words chosen.

As they grow older and acquire an increasing vocabulary, so too will children be more likely to comprehend a wider range of verbal communication. It cannot, however, be dissociated from the non-verbal signals, however sophisticated the linguistic content. The child responds to all the stimuli conveyed: tactile, visual and verbal.

The adult has to remain aware of the level of understanding a particular child has. Not only does this apply to the superficial meaning of words but also to the intrinsic abstract concepts which are being communicated.

Age is not the sole determinant of the level of understanding of a child. Other factors in the child's environment are equally important. The child's ability to understand is greatly influenced by how adults relate to him in all forms of communication. Psycholinguists suggest that the ability to understand abstract concepts is enhanced if adults, when communicating orally, do so using a broad range of both language and imagery to establish meaning.

THE CHILD-CENTRED APPROACH

How, therefore, does the adult determine the child's level of understanding either to communicate directly, for a variety of reasons, or as part of an assessment of development progress? The logical answer is to ask the child, or more accurately, allow the child to be the informant. This should set the level of communication on the child's terms, allowing the practitioner the chance to establish a rapport without either being patronising or talking 'over the child's head'. The shortest route to this is usually through play. If the child is allowed to play freely, the play will soon indicate the child's level of understanding and the practitioner can be guided by this to begin to establish a rapport.

Eye contact is vital and adults should ensure that they put themselves at the child's physical level whenever possible. Communication can be opened by asking the child to talk about his play. The simple request to 'tell me about it' suggests to the child that the adult is interested in the child and wants to know more about the child. This helps to make the child feel at ease. If the child is making a model or a picture, asking to have it explained is less patronising and more productive than saying 'That's good. What is it?'

When play or being on the child's level is not possible, a better rapport can still be achieved by bringing the child to the adult's level, such as sitting the child at a desk, or on the carer's knee, or on a high stool.

Conversation can begin with a few simple questions about, for example, the child's favourite toy, or food, or what the child likes to do. If the child is too young to talk, a small toy or paper and pencil for drawing can be effective means of communicating. This can reveal the child's perception of time and space, and establish the child's level of verbal understanding. Practitioners can then explore what they need to know in more depth. It has to be said that, too often, adults approach children in a way which is unproductive. If the child does not have confidence in the adult the potential for miscommunication is increased considerably.

When the child is older and play is perhaps less appropriate, similar principles to those described above apply. Adolescents tend to prefer an approach which is direct while not being intrusive, particularly if they have only just met the adult. They rarely appreciate being spoken down to, or adults who attempt to use adolescent-style idioms.

COMMUNICATION DIFFICULTIES

Communication may be more difficult when the adult or child has a communication disability, or a different mother tongue. Practitioners who have experience of children with communication disabilities or learning difficulties are usually able to develop alternate means of mutual understanding. If practitioners do not have the specialist knowledge required, it may be advantageous to enlist the help of colleagues who do. Non-verbal communication is an essential element of human interaction and when direct verbal communication is limited it is more necessary to use non-verbal techniques effectively. Equally, when a child has a visual disability, special care is needed to ensure purposeful communication.

When English is not the first language of the child or his parents, extra care should be taken to ensure mutual understanding. An incremental approach to establish the perceptions of a child and her family is useful. While an individual's vocabulary may be extensive, the hidden meanings in language may not always be fully understood. This could lead, for example, to a misinterpretation of symptoms or of the family's attitude towards the practitioner. Where possible, if there is uncertainty, it is useful to check with a colleague from the same culture and language base.

THE ROLE OF THE GUARDIAN AD LITEM

If a local authority makes an application to the courts in respect of a child, a guardian ad litem will, in most circumstances, be appointed to represent the child's interests [1]. The guardian will probably approach the child's medical practitioner to obtain an opinion concerning general health. In some circumstances the guardian may request that the practitioner examines the child in order to assess the child's current state of health and development.

Whatever the circumstances, the guardian will want to be satisfied that consent to examination has been given by the child and his parents. The child, if of an age to have sufficient understanding, should have given consent to the examination only after having been given all the relevant information. The parents' consent should also be sought. If the child is not of sufficient understanding, the guardian will want to know how well the parents have been appraised so their informed consent is given. The guardian will need to be satisfied that whatever the child's age, communication has been as clear and sympathetic as possible. A practitioner, in discussing the situation with the guardian, should be able to explain how he communicated with the child, what was said and what the child's responses were.

If the courts require a medical opinion, the practitioner will be able to report in the knowledge that the child has been as fully involved as possible in the process. This should not only give the practitioner confidence in the diagnosis or opinion but will also ensure that the child's welfare has been the paramount consideration.

THE *GILLICK* JUDGMENT

The implications of the *Gillick* judgment [2] are far greater than the specific issue of a child's right to confidentiality when seeking advice on contraception when under the age of 16. As well as clarifying the issue that parents have responsibility for, and not rights over, children, the judgment highlights the principle of 'sufficient understanding'. This means that all children should be as involved as possible in decisions which affect their health or welfare. If a child is of an age to understand sufficiently what is happening, not only should the child be consulted but also his views must be taken into account. This leads to the principle that the older a child is the more involvement he should have in determining decisions about himself. Practitioners, being aware of this, will wish to communicate in a manner which the child can understand and reflect on. Even very young children will be more at ease if such an atmosphere exists and are less likely to be distressed by examinations. Parents will also be more relaxed and their non-verbal communication to the child will be more positive.

SUSPICIONS OF SEXUAL ABUSE

A practitioner may be concerned that a child is the victim of sexual abuse. Medical or behavioural symptoms, or a disclosure made directly to the practitioner, may suggest this.

If a parent expresses concern, the practitioner may wish to make an examination. The child protection procedures are explicit that any investigative examination in cases of suspected sexual abuse should be carried out by specially trained police surgeons and paediatricians, usually after an investigative interview by a social worker and police officer [3]. The role of the general practitioner in such cases is to make a referral to social services so that an investigation can be initiated. Both child and parent will want to be assured that the appropriate action will be taken, and clear, sympathetic communication should take place.

Older children, who may have spoken directly to their doctor, will need reassurance and an empathetic response. However difficult the child's story is to accept, perhaps due to its bizarre nature or a knowledge of the alleged perpetrator, the child should feel that his account is being taken seriously and will be investigated. Non-verbal responses are important at this time, as negative body language will be communicated as clearly as the spoken word. The child has vested trust in the practitioner and this should be respected. Children should be told that their disclosure cannot be a secret and evidence may have to be given in court.

CONCLUSION

Communication with children and adolescents is not always easy and good communication is not always possible. However, like many aspects of best practice in child care, it is a matter of being open, honest and clear. An unaffected, relaxed approach to children and their parents will not only ease stressful situations but will also yield results and confidence in the practitioner.

The fundamental philosophy of the Act, that the welfare of the child is paramount, is achieved in partnership with parents.

In contested cases, courts and guardians ad litem will be more likely to be persuaded that a diagnostic opinion is accurate when it is clear that steps have been taken to relate fully to both child and parent.

Recently, a survivor of sexual abuse, when asked why she had not told anybody at the time, replied 'because I didn't know anybody I thought would listen to me'.

REFERENCES

1. Children Act 1989, s 41
2. *Gillick v West Norfolk and Wisbech Area Health Authority and Another* [1986] AC 112, [1986] 1 FLR 224, discussed in Chapter 10
3. See local Area Child Protection Committee Inter-Agency Child Protection Procedures

Chapter 12

INTER-AGENCY CO-OPERATION IN THE INVESTIGATION OF CHILD ABUSE

INTRODUCTION

The protection of children from abuse and exploitation is a responsibility of all capable adults in the community. Practitioners who work with children are guided by their professional associations. These associations advise their members that their first responsibility is to the child when abuse, or potential abuse, is suspected. The Act is clear in its intention that agencies should co-operate in the investigation of suspected child abuse; this being in the best interest of the child.

The Act places the prime duty for investigations of child abuse with the local authority, the emphasis being to establish whether the child is suffering, or is likely to suffer, significant harm. The local authority shall make, or cause to be made, such inquiries as it considers necessary to enable it to decide whether it should take any action to safeguard or promote the child's welfare.

The Act further states [1] that other agencies have a duty to assist the local authority as and when appropriate. The National Health Services Act requires that health authorities and local authorities co-operate in exercising their respective functions. Health authorities must comply with requests for help from local authorities when this does not conflict with the discharge of their own duties [2].

In essence, this means that there is a statutory and professional expectation of inter-agency co-operation in all investigations of child abuse. Although this may seem all too obvious, numerous inquiries into child deaths since the death of Maria Colwell in 1974 have indicated a breakdown in co-operation between agencies. The report into the Cleveland affair [3] highlighted how inter-agency working can easily become dysfunctional when agencies disagree over particular issues surrounding investigations. It most vividly illustrated that it is the children who suffer the ramifications of these disagreements and withdrawal of co-operation.

WORKING TOGETHER

The Department of Health publication *Working Together – a Guide to Arrangements for Inter-agency Cooperation for the Protection of Children from Abuse* was revised in 1991 [4] to take into account the provisions of the Act. Its title underlines the department's commitment towards inter-agency co-operation. Practitioners are advised to read this document. It emphasises the process of co-operation reinforced by statute.

AREA CHILD PROTECTION COMMITTEES AND PROCEDURES

The role of the Area Child Protection Committee (ACPC) is to oversee inter-agency child protection policy and practice within a geographical area, usually that covered by the local social services department and the district health authority. Membership includes representatives of each agency who are of sufficient seniority to speak on their agency's behalf. This will include social service departments, police, medical practi tioners including general practitioners, community health workers, probation, education, child health, and any other agency which has a significant involvement in protecting children who may be at risk.

Each agency is responsible for the coordination of child protection policy and practice among their own personnel, which may include the production and distribution of child protection procedures. These should be based on the principles laid down in the inter-agency child protection procedures issued by ACPCs. Practitioners should ensure that they have access to these inter-agency procedures. Procedures should incorporate the philosophy and detail of the Act with particular emphasis on the paramountcy of the child's interests, working in partnership with parents and inter-agency co-operation.

TRAINING IN INTER-AGENCY CO-OPERATION

The inquiry into the death of Liam Johnson [5] recommended that all ACPCs ensure that inter-disciplinary training is treated as a priority.

This now happens in many areas and practitioners are advised to participate. Participation is doubly advantageous as delegates can inform colleagues from other disciplines as to relevant factors which will affect their practice, as well as professionally benefiting themselves from interaction with a variety of associates from other specialisms. Working together is something most professionals aim to do, and as it is now a fundamental principle of the Act, all practitioners have a duty and responsibility to promote it as a principle.

THE INITIAL PROCESS OF INVESTIGATIONS

When any person suspects or knows about child abuse, they should report this as soon as possible. Lay people may first refer their concerns to social services, the police, the NSPCC, a school, or want to talk to their general practitioner, health visitor or any person of authority.

The referrer should be advised that it is in the child's best interests that they talk directly to social services. If they find this too difficult, they may be able to overcome their reticence by discussion. If not, practitioners should make a detailed referral to social services. It is often very difficult for people to express their fears for a child formally, especially if they fear retaliation from the adults concerned, or are worried about breaking up a family.

When the practitioner has initial suspicions, the referral should be as detailed as possible both in terms of the suspicion and background history. Referrals should be followed, or made, in writing. Detailed reports are an invaluable element of the inquiry and not subject to changes of perception or lapses of memory as a verbal report might be.

Practitioners are advised to have as much factual information available as possible: full names, dates of birth, address, siblings, family contact, race, religion, culture, any communication or language difficulties, schools, and other agencies involved. Practitioners may give their opinion about any perceived injury, but they should deal only with what they observe.

When practitioners have their own suspicions or direct observation of evidence of abuse, they should take great care to clarify what part they will be playing in any consequent investigation. Parents may want to talk to their general practitioner or health visitor, for example, and it should be made clear, tactfully, that an investigation will have to take place. An injury may be observed and the child's or adult's explanation may not be consistent, or contradictory, or change irrationally. Those adults concerned should be told calmly that the explanation is not consistent and social services will be contacted. It must be noted at this point that suspicions of child sexual abuse are investigated in a different way from other forms of abuse and it is not necessarily appropriate to discuss such suspicions with the parent at this stage. If a perpetrator believes he is under suspicion, or that the child may be diagnosed as having been abused, he may use a variety of tactics to silence the child and so perpetuate the sexual abuse.

Following the referral, social workers have to make inquiries. These are designed to establish if an investigation should be launched. Practitioners should be involved. Their knowledge of children and their families is invaluable and information they provide may establish that suspicions are unfounded, or that further investigation is needed. Practitioners often have background knowledge which is not available to other professionals but which is vital to inquiries.

In addition to obtaining factual information, practitioners may observe patterns of stress or behaviour which may give rise to concern about children living in particular families. This may be stress which could lead to direct physical abuse, or patterns of child care which constitute emotional abuse or neglect. Neglect, and particularly non-organic failure to thrive, is a diagnosis dependent on the expertise of practitioners.

PARTNERSHIP AND POSITIVE PROGRESS

It should be noted that, as part of their role, practitioners encourage the enhancement of parenting skills. This aspect of the relationship between practitioner and parents is an essential part of child protection not only because of its positive nature but also in the possible prevention of abuse and neglect by empowering parents with knowledge and confidence in their parenting abilities.

The culture of working in partnership with parents is enshrined in the spirit of the Act [6]. Therefore, when child abuse is being investigated, parents should be informed as to what is happening and where possible, involved in the process. It is often the case that concerns are more readily resolved when this atmosphere prevails. If parents understand that agencies are endeavouring to promote the best interests of their child, and that they are not condemning them as cruel, wicked, failures or inadequate, they are more likely to understand the need for positive progress, and work towards it.

The Rochdale Report [7] commented that all agencies should concentrate on the positive aspects of families in which abuse had occurred in order to enable them to progress. Past abuse should not, of course, be ignored, nor should it be allowed to dominate future thinking; moreover, parties should work together to encourage progress.

Working in partnership with parents for the best interests of the child should begin at the outset of contact with a family. The later the attempts to engage parents, the more problems there are likely to be. Child protection work should be a continuum, not incremental. The continuum can only advance if parties not only understand what each other is doing but also why they are doing it. It is work which is fraught with emotional difficulties for the child, parents and workers. A lack of understanding and co-operation between professionals can lead to difficulties and this will not serve the best interests of the child.

Co-operation can range from the straightforward exchange of information to direct involvement with the child and family. Each stage needs to be properly negotiated so that those coordinating the assessment can maintain an accurate overview. The foundation stone for this is the child protection conference.

CHILD PROTECTION CONFERENCES

The child protection conference exists to form a view about what has happened to a child, any level of potential risk, how agencies and families can best communicate and work together, and what can be done to alleviate future risk. It must be said that conferences are not a guarantee that a child will not be abused in the future, and conference members may have to acknowledge that a child remains with his family despite the risk of future abuse.

The conference, once fully informed by all parties, should agree recommended courses of action by the various parties. The essence of best practice in child protection is that actions are part of a co-ordinated protection plan involving both professionals and families. Individual practitioners should, therefore, understand that they will be working in partnership with colleagues and families. This should ensure that the process is not condemnatory of parents but child-centred with a view to assessing the nature of any abuse and treating its consequences in the short term, and preventing or diminishing abuse in the longer term.

The nature of child abuse is such that attempting to achieve an incremental decrease is often more realistic than immediate eradication. This is particularly relevant to emotional abuse, neglect and inappropriate chastisement. Clearly, once an investigation has established that a child is being, for example, sexually abused and who the perpetrator is, total prevention is the immediate aim. In order to assess the reality of each of these goals, the conference has to integrate a broad knowledge of the child's circumstances.

As parents have responsibilities, they have the right to be involved where possible and the responsibility to engender the best interests of their child. Consequently, in practice, parents should attend child protection conferences. Most children remain in their homes after they have been abused; or if accommodated or looked after in care they return home – permanent separation being relatively unusual. If parents attend conferences which are attempting to support the family, it is hoped that they will react more positively to advice. Since no adult likes to feel that they are perceived as having abused their child, changes in their attitude or behaviour are likely to be much greater if they are not alienated by the child protection agencies. Also, as a therapeutic tool, it is often beneficial that parents understand that concerns about their methods of child care are shared by a team of people and not by an individual practitioner who may appear to be vindictive or discriminatory.

The conference must be properly managed and parents should be encouraged to participate rather than just being in passive attendance. Conference members should be aware that most parents are not used to attending such meetings and are, therefore, at a disadvantage. Conferences are not part of the judicial process and should not, therefore, set themselves the task of proving guilt or innocence. The role of the conference is to promote the best interests of the child and to endeavour to prevent further abuse. Parents should not be harangued, accused, threatened or pressurised into agreeing to act in a way which is unreasonable, or to achieve impossible goals.

Parents may be from minority ethnic groups, from different cultural backgrounds, be disabled or have communication difficulties, be single parents, come from a different class to the professionals, not have English as a first language, be mentally vulnerable, or perhaps under considerable stress due to economic deprivation or sub-standard housing. In such cases, regardless of the nature of the disadvantage, the conference should be properly chaired and members should behave in a way which does not discriminate against parents and which positively encourages parents to see themselves as having a valuable role in their child's life.

Concerns and views about potential resolutions should be made in a clear, non-jargonistic, non-condemnatory manner. Practitioners should not make value judgments but base their assessments on the collective information gathered. The person chairing the conference should ensure that the views of participants are based on conference content, not on unreported information, rumour, local gossip, or any of the numerous unspoken influences which may improperly prejudice decision-making.

As the Act dictates that the child's interests are paramount and that statutory intervention should only be initiated when not doing so would be more harmful to the child, the conference members should try to adopt this approach. How can the child's safety be maintained while investing as much responsibility as possible in the child's parent? The child protection plan, if inappropriately implemented, may invest too much responsibility in the professionals while leaving care to the parent. This is unsatisfactory for everyone and is likely to mean that the child's best interests are not served.

THE PRACTITIONER AS SPECIALIST

Each practitioner will have his or her own area of specialism which should be maximised in the investigation. Specialisms may range from the broad knowledge of the general practitioner to the more specific, such as dermatology, psychiatry or venereology. Para-medical practitioners will have their own areas of expertise, such as health education. Individuals should not undervalue their potential contribution and each particular investigation should include as wide a variety of specialist inputs as possible.

As difficulties can arise in agreeing a diagnosis, no single practitioner should assume that his is the only correct diagnosis, or be professionally offended when a particular alternative specialist opinion is sought.

Practitioners should receive training in the signs and symptoms of child abuse from an appropriately experienced specialist, such as a consultant paediatrician. Training should alert practitioners to basic symptomology and so inform their practice when they are examining children. Practitioners, as members of a primary health team, may have a number of concerns because of background knowledge of a family, whereas, for example, orthopaedists or dentists may have little information other than the presentation of a particular injury or symptom. They may have the expertise to make judgments about cause and effect from direct observation and information received as to how an injury occurred, but all practitioners need to be aware of the likelihood of child abuse and the expectation that they contribute to, or initiate, inter-agency investigations.

THE INVESTIGATION OF SEXUAL ABUSE

Child sexual abuse investigations can be almost as traumatic to a child as the abuse itself, and because of this and the fact that the perpetrators of the abuse may silence the child, careful planning is needed before the investigation takes place.

Practitioners may be approached by anxious parents or colleagues who are disturbed by a child's behaviour or alarmed by particular symptoms which they have observed themselves. However, if they become concerned, or if a child wishes to disclose information about abuse, it should be made clear that that information will be passed to social services. Agreement to keep confidences may lead to being trapped in the same web of secrecy as the victims and thus, unintentionally, encourage the continuation of the abuse.

An investigative interview by a police officer and a social worker will usually take place and this will be video taped. If this establishes likely abuse a medical examination will then be arranged. This should be done jointly by a police surgeon and consultant paediatrician. They may request that other practitioners provide them with information about the child in order to facilitate the investigation. As it is a forensic examination the results may be used in legal proceedings, either criminal or civil. Children should only be examined once, as the examination is physically intrusive and likely to be traumatic.

In cases of sexual abuse, urgent medical intervention should take place only: if there has been a recent sexual act and evidence has been found such as semen; if the child has sustained physical injuries which necessitate urgent medical assistance; if the perpetrator is likely to abscond and evidence will secure his arrest and detention or if the child requests immediate treatment.

Where possible, investigators should involve the non-abusing parent or carer at the earliest stages. Knowing that a child has been sexually abused can be very difficult for any parent to accept and if the professionals do not involve the non-abusing parent it is possible that that parent will deny any abuse has occurred and may then be wrongly accused of colluding with the perpetrator. This can lead to the inappropriate removal of the child, rather than the perpetrator, from the family. The Act recognises this and allows local authorities to provide resources so that suspected perpetrators can move from their family homes [8]. It is in the interests of all parties that practitioners and local social workers establish relationships which allow for general, as well as specific, discussions of worries they may have about children. When appropriate, specific referrals can then be made in an atmosphere of co-operation and understanding of each other's professional philosophy.

The non-abusing carer is likely to be traumatised by the fact that someone in or close to the family has sexually abused a child of the family. There may be feelings of guilt and anger, and signs of extreme stress. Practitioners can be highly supportive at this time. Reassurance and support will help promote the rebuilding of family life. A non-condemnatory approach is vital as there is likely to be guilt at the failure to prevent the abuse, particularly if the non-abuser feels responsible for bringing the perpetrator into the home; or having been accused by the perpetrator of failing to satisfy his sexual needs, believes that this forced the perpetrator to turn on the child. Perpetrators of sexual abuse will often try to excuse their actions by this, or other, explanations. The reality is that they have abused their power as adults over children and they alone are responsible. In most instances, however, the perpetrator is devious in his activity and carries out the abuse usually without the knowledge or consent of the non-abusing parent.

If children are sexually abused by other children, the method of investigation will generally be the same. However, care will also be paid to the alleged abuser as he may well be being abused himself, or have experienced abuse. When organised abuse, by a number of adults, is suspected, the investigations are more complex and will not only involve specialist planning but may take considerable time and resources. Practitioners may have to deal with the stress on families caused by this. In whatever manner a child has been abused, that child will want and need assurance on several matters: that they have not been permanently damaged physically or emotionally, that they have not contracted a sexually transmitted disease, that they are not mad or bad, and perhaps most importantly, that they are not to blame. How each of these matters is dealt with by the practitioners will depend upon the age of the child and the nature of any injuries or infections. If specialist treatment is needed, following forensic examination, this will need to be discussed with the child and the non-abusing parent with a great deal of circumspection. It may also be appropriate, or requested, that counselling be offered about HIV/AIDS.

Psychosomatic symptoms in a child could indicate not only distress or disturbance but also abuse. Perpetrators often ensnare children by secrecy and threat, projecting the guilt for the activity onto the child. Threats may be made to physically injure, or even kill, the child, the mother, the siblings or the family pet. However the child is silenced, it could lead to that child presenting with behavioural problems. Disturbed sleep patterns, nightmares, stomach pains, headaches, withdrawal, indiscriminate chattering; whatever the symptoms, practitioners should not ignore the possibility of sexual abuse. A parent or teacher may be worried that a child is inappropriately masturbating, or has contracted a genital infection from no apparent source. Concern about such symptoms should be referred to social services. Practitioners may wish to discuss a child or family with colleagues from community child health services, the consultant community paediatrician, the hospital consultant paediatrician or senior clinical medical officer. They will also be advised that social services must be involved.

Practitioners and social workers should establish relationships so that concerns can be discussed and, when appropriate, referrals made. Involving a third party is less satisfactory, and practitioners should not request others to make a referral on their behalf unless it is unavoidable.

Investigations into sexual abuse should always take gender, race, culture and religion into account.

OTHER FORMS OF CHILD ABUSE

Public and professional attention has been focused most notably in the past on physical abuse and more recently on sexual abuse. Many children are subject, however, to emotional abuse or neglect. All child abuse contains elements of emotional abuse, but this may be the prevailing behaviour of an adult towards a child.

Emotional abuse can range from the frequent belittling of a child to what may be described as mental torture. Practitioners may have experience of direct observation of such abuse, or the symptoms which arise from it. Emotional abuse may be difficult to measure scientifically but the long-term effects on the mental well-being of a child can be devastating. Discussions with specialist colleagues can be invaluable and therapeutic intervention can help the child.

Neglect can also be hard to quantify. It can be damaging physically, emotionally and environmentally, causing serious impairment to health and development. Neglect can range from leaving the child alone and vulnerable to accident, exploitation or injury, to failure to attend to the child's physical and developmental well-being. Non-organic failure to thrive may result from the neglect of a child and always requires medical diagnosis.

Health education plays an important role in child care to help develop a positive, co-operative atmosphere. Professionals can proactively address potential neglect by engendering awareness of children's needs. When neglect is diagnosed, the health education aspects of a practitioner's role can come to the fore in advising and guiding parents as to their child's needs.

INSTITUTIONAL CHILD ABUSE

When institutions fail to meet the needs of the child, this, too, can be defined as abuse of a child. For example:

(a) inappropriate removal from families;
(b) repeated intrusive interviews or examinations;
(c) failure to admit abuse is taking place;
(d) non-referral of suspicions;
(e) non-acceptance of responsibility for the child's welfare;
(f) allowing inter-professional disagreements or disputes to cloud judgment or prevent co-operation;
(g) inappropriate negative labelling of families;
(h) a lack of honesty and directness with children and parents;
(i) the engendering of discrimination due to race, culture, religion, gender, disability or sexuality.

All practitioners have a duty to avoid such abuse and address it as soon as it becomes apparent.

RACE, CULTURE, RELIGION, CLASS, DISABILITY, GENDER AND SEXUALITY

Views about good child care vary among families, races, cultures, creeds and classes. No single model of family life is correct and different views should not compete with each other. Practitioners should take this into account when assessing families. The Act is specific that a child's racial and religious needs are taken into account [9].

Child abuse exists in all communities yet no society finds the abuse of children acceptable. Practitioners should be wary of over-critical views of families from other races and cultures; conversely they should not over-compensate for abusive behaviour, assuming that it is culturally appropriate. If practitioners are unsure of cultural parenting patterns, they are advised to consult with colleagues from the same ethnic or cultural background as the family concerned.

If English is not the first language of a family, the practitioner should ensure that the family understands what is being said, what expectations there are of the parenting role, and that the parents understand their rights and responsibilities. The co-operative aspects of child protection work should promote understanding and a positive awareness of differences.

Mental or physical disability in a family may be a contributory stress factor in a few cases of child abuse. Communication difficulties and the disability of a child is not a mitigator against abuse; where on the one hand recent investigations have shown that disabled children may be particularly vulnerable to exploitation and abuse from non-family members, on the other hand many adults with disabilities have children and their ability as parents is not in doubt.

Gender is a vital factor in child protection. Practitioners not only need to be aware that a gender difference can radically affect relationships but also that great care has to be taken over the gender of investigators when there is suspected abuse, especially sexual abuse.

Many cultures have specific conventions about gender roles and the behaviour between members of either sex. These will strongly influence, for example, communication or perceived attitudes towards authority.

The vast majority of perpetrators of sexual abuse are men [10] and this abuse of their power over children is likely to affect the survivor's view of all men, certainly when the abuse is recent. Investigators should be very mindful of this and children should not be interviewed or medically examined solely by men. A child who has been abused will most probably find a medical examination to be intrusive. In some cases, consideration may have to be given to excluding male professionals from particular aspects of an investigation.

Where a parent is homosexual, assumptions should not be made about their parenting abilities. Similarly, negative presuppositions should not be made about single parents, of either sex. It should be noted here, however, that the majority of sexual abusers are heterosexual males [11] and that those people who physically or emotionally abuse or neglect their children come from all sectors of society.

Assumptions should also not be made about black and minority ethnic families, or parents and children from minority and disadvantaged groups. Being aware of the need not to make assumptions in all circumstances is the best practice. Awareness should ensure a more objective approach to all investigations and that conclusions about families do not come from negative stereotypes, but from shared information and knowledge.

STATUTORY INTERVENTION

Parts IV and V of the Act relate to the public law on the need to prevent children from suffering or potentially suffering significant harm. Part IV relates to the longer-term intervention of supervision and care orders, whereas Part V refers to the shorter-term need to protect children at risk by emergency intervention by the courts. The detail of the various elements of Parts IV and V is dealt with in other parts of this book. It is sufficient to note here that when the courts are involved, any decision which they make is most likely to be in the child's best interests when all parties have worked together.

CONCLUSION

The successful investigation of abuse depends on inter-agency co-operation. Practitioners should be aware of their statutory and procedural responsibilities as well as the importance of their specialism to the child. Child protection is stressful and complex and children can too easily suffer when adults disagree. Procedures [12] exist which should allow for conciliation between parties when problems arise. No professional should criticise the ability of parents to co-operate if they themselves are not able to work in partnership with their colleagues. Failure to do so is a failure of their duty to protect a child.

REFERENCES

1. Children Act 1989, s 27
2. National Health Service Act 1977
3. *Report of the Inquiry into Child Abuse in Cleveland* (Cmnd 412, 1988)
4. *Working Together Under the Children Act* (HMSO, 1991)
5. *Report of the Enquiry into the Death of Liam Johnson* (Islington ACPC, 1990)
6. See DOH *Guidance* to the Act
7. Social Services Inspectorate *Report on Child Protection Services in Rochdale* (HMSO, 1991)
8. Children Act 1989, Sch 2, para 5
9. Children Act 1989, s 11(3)
10. Finkelhor D *Child Sexual Abuse* (Free Press, New York, 1984); for a full discussion see Glaser D and Frosh S *Child Sexual Abuse* (Macmillan, London, 1988) ch 1
11. Glaser D, ibid
12. See local Area Child Protection Committee Inter-Agency Child Protection Procedures

Chapter 13

PREPARATION OF REPORTS FOR COURT

Many expert witnesses are asked to prepare a report for court proceedings and, if the report is accepted in evidence by the court and the other parties to the case, they may not then be required to attend court personally to give oral evidence. If a report is well prepared and clear, it has a better chance of being accepted as it stands. However, in many cases attendance at court is inevitable. Where scientific or medical issues are disputed, that evidence will usually be tested by cross-examination. Chapter 14 looks at preparation for attendance at court and developing courtroom skills.

Good preparation adds more cogency and authority to a report than its physical presentation in court by the witness. However well written, the evidential value of a report increases in almost direct proportion to the degree of accuracy and clarity of its terminology and the preparation of the material on which it is based. Below are a few ideas that may be of some assistance.

NOTES AND RECORDS

Most reports, of whatever kind, will be prepared using records and notes made or kept by the expert witness. If a conclusion results from information drawn from personal observations, dialogue, or from others' observations, that conclusion must be capable of justification by the person stating it. It is difficult for those who see many patients or clients to remember details of all relevant information, and so notes and records are vital. A practitioner may, for example, need to refer to the notes made by colleagues or staff. Notes, therefore, have to be clear, accurate, dated, and accessible. It is a common occurrence that a doctor may be asked to give a medical report of a patient who has attended the surgery or hospital several times and perhaps seen other practitioners who have each added to the notes on the patient's record. The report will be based upon the notes of others as well as those of the writer of the report. Where this occurs it should be acknowledged in the report, which should clearly indicate which events involved the witness personally, and which did not. It may sometimes be necessary, if detail is required of a specific recorded incident (for example, of conversation remembered by the patient but not entered by the practitioner in the notes), to call the practitioner involved on that occasion as a witness.

Notes forming part of a continuous record (such as a patient record) are, for the purposes of court proceedings, admissible in evidence even if each contributor to those notes is not there to present his contribution personally. This is a rule of necessity because practitioners frequently move with their jobs, and it is quite often necessary to refer to the notes made by a predecessor. Bearing in mind that any notes might end up in court in one way or another, it is wise to be careful about the choice of words used to ensure accuracy and clarity. Also, if personal reactions to a particular individual are strong, and there is a temptation to record them, it is useful to consider first whether one's judgment is justifiable and whether that judgment is subjective. We all have prejudices of one sort or another and it is helpful to identify and acknowledge them. In this way, discrimination of any sort can be tackled. Also, this means that if a witness is asked in court to explain any personal comment appearing in notes or a report, that witness will be better able to do so.

As notes may become vital evidence, they should not be subsequently deleted to make corrections. Additions may be made to correct facts which have for any reason been incorrectly recorded earlier. Such additions should be in the form of an addendum, leaving the original wording intact and clearly legible, and the addendum should be acknowledged, signed and dated by the person making it. If possible, there should be an explanation of how the fact was incorrectly recorded, how it came to be noticed, and an acknowledgment of responsibility by the person(s) involved. Obviously, a mistake in the record of medication or treatment given, or of a finding in an examination, could be as vital in a court case as it is in patient care, and so careful, accurate record-keeping is essential.

PREPARATION

Before starting to write a report, make sure that all the relevant information is available – notes, records, charts, graphs, X-rays, and any other data which are relevant to the issues. If references are to be used, they need to be accurately quoted and cited. It is hoped that there will have been good background information as to the circumstances of the case provided by the party requesting the report, and there may have been earlier reports by other experts in the same case. All of these may be needed in the preparation of a comprehensive report to the court. Logical sequencing of thought is important, and the report should be carefully structured. There are many ways of structuring a report, and the needs of individual cases will dictate the content of reports but, generally, the ideas set out below may prove useful.

FORMAT OF MEDICAL REPORTS FOR COURT

Children Act 1989 Reports/Statements

The Rules made pursuant to the Children Act 1989 [1] provide that in cases under the Act, the party calling a witness must file with the court and serve on other parties a written statement of the substance of the oral evidence which the party intends to call at the proceedings [2].

These statements must be dated, signed by the person making the statement, and contain a declaration that the maker of the statement believes it to be true and understands that it may be placed before the court [3]. Any research, reports or documents to be relied upon by that witness should be referred to in the report and, if possible, copies attached. Supplementary statements may be filed, subject to the directions of the court.

There is a prohibition on medical or psychiatric examination or assessment of a child for the purpose of expert evidence in court proceedings without the leave of the court [4].

Format of Children Act 1989 Report/Statement

Head the report in a way which identifies the court and the proceedings for which the statement is intended.

'In the .... Court

Case Reference No ....

Proceedings ....

Re (*name of child(ren) and date of birth*)....................................

NB. Do *not* include address of child unless authorised to do so (see Confidentiality below at p 110).

Report of Dr...

Date...'
CONFIDENTIAL

The text should follow a logical sequence, with numbered paragraphs, each containing a relevant point. This makes it easier to refer to the statement in court.

The final paragraph should be worded to comply with the requirements of the Rules [5].

'I .... (Full name) .... declare that the content of this my statement is true to the best of my knowledge, information, and belief; and I understand that this statement may be placed before the court.

Signed ....

Dated ....

Freda Smith MD'

Affidavits in Civil, Non-Children Act Proceedings

The good news is that affidavits are *not* required for proceedings under the Children Act 1989. However, affidavits are still required for non-Children Act cases in the county court and High Court, so there is included here a short account of affidavit format and procedure.

An affidavit is the name given to the document of written evidence traditionally designed for use in the High Court and the county court, following a specific format and then sworn or affirmed as the truth by the deponent. Attached to an affidavit may be other documents which support its content; these are referred to as 'exhibits'. Each exhibit must be clearly labelled and identified. Usually, expert witnesses are not expected to know all these finer details, and reports submitted for these courts are put where necessary into affidavit form by the solicitor for the party instructing them, then sent back to the expert to be sworn or affirmed.

Format for Affidavits

Each affidavit should be appropriately headed indicating the court in which the action is taking place, the court reference number and the parties to the action. There usually follows, beneath this, a title indicating who the person is making it, for example 'Affidavit of Jane Smith'. The document is designed with an outer cover bearing the same headings and also the name and address of the party filing it.

The body of the text traditionally begins like this:

'I .... (full name) .... of (address) ....
MAKE OATH and say as follows:'

or, if the deponent objects to taking an oath, then

'I .... (full name) .... of (address) ....
DO SOLEMNLY DECLARE AND AFFIRM as follows:'

The text should follow in numbered paragraphs, each following a logical order, containing one of the points the deponent wishes to make. This makes it easier to refer to the affidavit in court, for the judge, the parties, and the witness.

At the end of the affidavit comes the Jurat, or the Affirmation:

'Sworn at .... (or Declared at)
in the County of ....
This .... day of .... 19..
Before me ....
Solicitor/Commissioner for Oaths'

The affidavit has then to be taken to a solicitor or a commissioner for oaths, and sworn or declared to be true. Nominated members of the county court and High Court staff will also administer oaths and affirmations. A fee is chargeable for each affidavit and exhibit sworn.

CONTENT OF REPORTS GENERALLY

Headings

The heading should follow the format for Children Act 1989 Reports/ Statements outlined above on pp 101–2.

Personal Information

The report would usually begin with the following information:

- practitioner's name;
- practising address;
- work telephone number (and facsimile number, DX, etc);
- professional position or appointments held;
- qualifications;
- relevant experience.

(Here, wide experience in another field may be impressive in general terms but will have little influence on the court. Relevant experience, which could lend greater authority to judgments and evaluations, is frequently left out, and could be usefully included.)

Events Leading to Conclusions Drawn, with Dates where Relevant

Where an assertion is made in a report, the basis upon which the assertion is made should be clear. Failure to state the observations leading to a conclusion could well cause adverse comment in court, exposing the expert to criticism of method or judgment. A judgment made after several long interviews with someone may well carry more weight than one based upon a quick once-only meeting. It is necessary to let the court know these details. Dates are usually highly relevant. The last interview or examination may have preceded a change in circumstances, altering the outlook of the case. It is advisable to have the complete file of documents and correspondence, notes, or papers to hand in court for reference. Without these, it is possible to be caught out on minor technicalities, leaving the court with an impression of disorganisation or even incompetence.

Sources of Information

It helps to keep a note of information sources for personal reference when preparing a report. This could include:

- names of persons interviewed;
- number of interviews of each person;
- dates and frequency/spacing of interviews which may be relevant. Were any appointments missed? Why?;
- where relevant, circumstances and venue of interviews and any examinations carried out;
- places visited eg home, school, relatives' homes;
- samples examined;
- any other examinations or assessments made, etc, which are relevant to the issues.

In many cases, children often relax in the safety of hospital or foster care, and begin to say things which may be relevant to those they trust. Staff should be encouraged to note carefully any comments or actions which they think may be important to the case. Changes in behaviour should be noted as they are often significant.

Chronology/Diary Entries

It is difficult in a complex case for the court or anyone else to hold in mind the full sequence of events. The chronology (which is usually prepared by the applicant or his or her solicitor, often the local authority) is a list of the most important and relevant events in the child's life together with action taken including any court orders made, set out in chronological order, with appropriate dates, and usually proves invaluable. Practitioners may ask for a copy of the chronology, or have their own diary of medical events to assist them in preparation of their report.

Account of Questioning and Information Leading to Observations and Conclusions

Conversation with a child, or anyone else, may contain information relevant to the issues before the court. If conversation is recorded in notes, or recalled from memory, it should form part of the report where reliance is placed upon it as evidence leading to a conclusion.

The Act gives a child the right to make an informed refusal of medical or psychiatric assessment or examination in certain circumstances (see Chapter 10). The doctor concerned and the guardian ad litem may be asked to advise the court as to the ability of the child to make an informed decision. It is vital to record the conversation which takes place around this issue. A child cannot make an 'informed decision' without being given adequate information which is appropriate to his age and understanding, and the report may need to set out the substance of the information provided for the child. Questions eliciting the child's response to the examination and to any other issues in the case could be vitally important and should be noted, together with the child's responses.

Illustrations and Photographs

Sketches of the body indicating sites of injury, or any other record made by the practitioner at the time of an examination or immediately afterwards may be used in evidence and annexed to a report or statement. Photographs of injuries, scan results and X-rays may be tendered in evidence. The person who took them should produce them formally, either by bringing them to court, or attaching them as exhibits to a statement, with a rider to the effect that that person took the photograph and that the unretouched negative is in his or her possession. If they form part of a hospital record they may be produced as part of that record. On the question of ownership and storage, they belong to the hospital. In general law, a photograph belongs to the person who owns the film unless it is specially commissioned with a different contractual arrangement between photographer and client.

The ownership of the photograph does not affect its legal validity as evidence. If, for example, an X-ray is produced as part of a continuous hospital record, by a person other than the person who actually took the X-ray, it may be allowed in evidence, but there could be limitations on the ability of the person at court to make observations about it if they were not present at the time the X-ray was taken.

Exhibits

Relevant evidence may include other material, or objects which the court will refer to as 'exhibits'. For example, a report might wish to refer to a document, an object, a photograph or a video or tape-recording.

Documents

If a document is essential to a case, either the original or a copy of it should be attached to the court report or affidavit. The court prefers to have the original if this is possible, but if the original forms part of a continuous record, and cannot be spared for court use, a copy of the relevant part (duly certified by the person making the report writing at the top of the copy 'I have compared this with the original, and certify it to be a true copy', signed .... dated ....) should be attached to the report together with a note confirming that the original will be brought to court by the witness for inspection at the hearing, or will be made available for inspection.

Medical records are confidential and should not be annexed to reports for court unless the practitioner is satisfied that: (a) necessary consents for disclosure have been obtained; and (b) disclosure will not harm the patient; and (c) the information is vital to the case and is required by the court.

The directions of the court should always be sought if the practitioner has any doubts about disclosure of information or any document. (See Chapter 10 and Appendix 1 on confidentiality and consent.)

If the exhibit is a document, it is courteous to make sufficient copies for the court (in the family proceedings court, four are required – one for each magistrate and one for the clerk to the court) and copies for each party to the case, the guardian ad litem, and any other experts. The rules provide that statements shall be served in advance upon the court and the other parties [6], and the technicalities of service and copying will usually be dealt with by the solicitor who is calling the expert witness.

Objects

Any object which is vital to the evidence must be brought to court or be available for inspection. The court will usually want to keep the object during the proceedings. Body samples, fibres, toxic substances and other materials found in forensic investigation are, of course, often produced to the courts. The court will go and 'view' objects and scenes if absolutely necessary.

Photographs, Illustrations and X-rays

Where photographs are to be exhibited, the report must indicate who took them, and who holds the unretouched negatives. The court will want assurance that the negatives have not been tampered with. A photograph is best exhibited by the person who took it, or at least someone who was present when it was taken. Evidence may be required as to the date and conditions in which the photographs were taken. The negatives should be brought to court, or be readily available for inspection if the witness is not required to give oral evidence.

Audio and Video-tape Recordings

Tape recordings and video recordings are regarded in law as 'documents'.

When an incident is recorded as it is happening, for example a video recording of sexual activity with a child by someone who was present, this will be 'real evidence', which can be admitted both in criminal or civil cases. There is insufficient space here to go very far into the law of evidence, but for those who want to do so there are some excellent books available [7]. The criminal law of evidence is stricter than civil law. The burden of proof is heavier in criminal cases. In a criminal case the alleged offence has to be proved 'beyond reasonable doubt'. In civil cases, including Children Act proceedings, the circumstances alleged must be proved on 'a balance of probabilities', meaning that it is more likely than not that the alleged events occurred.

The most likely form of tape recording to come before the court in Children Act cases is that of an interview with a child by members of a team investigating alleged abuse, in which a disclosure may be made. An audio or video-tape recording of a child talking about an event after it happened is regarded at present as 'hearsay' which may render it inadmissible in evidence in criminal prosecutions, although it will be admissible in most Children Act cases. Hearsay evidence given in connection with the upbringing, maintenance or welfare of a child is allowed in all civil proceedings before a High Court and a county court, and in family proceedings before a magistrates' court [8]. This includes cases brought under the Children Act 1989. Tape-recorded interviews of children are, therefore, admissible, but the weight given by the court to any disclosures made in them depends upon the skill and competence of the interviewer.

There are now changes in the law of evidence to admit video interviews in certain types of criminal cases involving child witnesses [9]. The skill of the interviewer can radically affect the evidential quality of such a video recording. The Home Office has also recently published a memorandum of good practice for video-recorded interviews of child witnesses in criminal proceedings [10].

References

Reports often refer to research carried out by the witness, or by others. Clear references should be made so that the court can identify which work is that of the witness, and which is the work of others. If any research is cited as authority for a statement, then the report of that research should be made available for the court to see. Publications referred to as authority for opinions in the report should be cited in the usual way, with the author, publisher and date. See Chapter 14 for more about giving evidence and reliance upon authorities.

Terminology/Avoidance of Jargon

Try to avoid medical or technical jargon. Remember how irritating it is to be confronted with too much legalese! Court proceedings should not, but usually do, involve power games of one sort or another. The court is the lawyers' territory. Lawyers conduct proceedings in their language and in accordance with their rules. The use of terms which they do not fully understand engenders frustration. The most effective reports explain what they want to get across simply and clearly, without exaggeration or embellishment. If technical terms are necessary, then also provide an explanation of their meaning. When an opinion is being proffered, for example as to causation, it is helpful to include in the report comment as to whether the events or symptoms observed are commonly occurring or are indicative of something unusual. In this way the causal link is clear, and the report has a better chance of being understood and accepted. If the witness is called to court, there is less likelihood of confusion over the important issues during cross-examination.

Summaries

It always helps to include a clear summary in a report. There may need to be a certain amount of minor repetition, but to have a final summary of the conclusions drawn, and recommendations made, with reasons clearly set out, is helpful for the court. If various options have been considered before the final conclusion is made, then each alternative should have been addressed in the body of the report, and the reasons for the final decision or opinion given. The report should make clear, where relevant, that all possible avenues have been explored. The decision reached and recorded in the summary will, therefore, be seen to be balanced and well thought out.

Confidentiality

Where there are child protection or adoption issues, the current where-abouts of the child may be confidential. Medical reports in normal circumstances might often begin with the name, address and date of birth of the child. Care should be taken to check on confidentiality before including in any report information which could identify the child's address or their carers' names. This includes information which could give clues identifying school, playgroups or day nursery attended.

Previous Reports

If this is the second or subsequent report on the same matter, the content of earlier reports should be borne in mind. To avoid confusion where earlier information, diagnosis or prognosis has altered, clear reference should be made to the earlier report and the changes indicated with reasons where appropriate.

Report Checklist

Name

Practising address

Work Tel. No. / Fax No. / DX

Professional position or appointments held

Qualifications

Practitioner's relevant experience

Confidentiality checked

List of persons interviewed, or consulted, in connection with the pre-paration of this report (including times, dates, location, frequency, etc where the practitioner considers this relevant).

List of places visited in the preparation of the report, with details where relevant.

List of samples taken for the preparation of the report, with details if relevant, of times samples taken, data attached to sample, etc.

Chronology – can be useful to get things in context.

Final check with diary and notes. Are the details of dates and times given in the report accurate?

Has any information been given out? Is it recorded in the report and, if not, should it be?

Does the report refer to quoted comment from any interviews? If so, is there a contemporaneous note, and is the report giving an accurate account of what the notes record?

If the report is based upon information provided by others, has this been made clear in the report, and does the report make clear the nature of the information given, its source, the weight given to it, and the extent to which it has been relied upon?

Does the report make clear the basis upon which opinion is given and conclusions are drawn?

Has jargon been avoided?

Where technical terminology is unavoidable, is it also explained in clear terms?

Is the thinking process in the report clear and well reasoned?

Have all possible alternative avenues been explored, and is this made clear in the report?

Are there specific legal requirements for this case? Have they been met? Does the case require discussion with the lawyer instructing the practitioner?

Are there specific legal requirements of format or content for this court report? Are they all fulfilled?

Have there been any other reports on this issue? If they differ in fact or opinion, is it appropriate to indicate those differences and the reasons for the new facts or conclusions now being expressed.

List of exhibits referred to in the report.

List of references cited, authorities quoted, or any other work relied upon in the report, with copies if appropriate attached as exhibits. (If not attached, they should be available if requested for reference when the witness goes to court.)

REFERENCES

1. Family Proceedings Rules 1991, SI 1991/1247 (for the High Court and the county court); Family Proceedings Courts (Children Act 1989) Rules 1991, SI 1991/1395 (for the magistrates' courts)
2. Ibid, r 4.17(1); r 17(1)
3. Ibid, r 4.17(1)(a)(iii); r 17(1)(a)(iii)
4. Ibid, r 4.18; r 18
5. Ibid, r 4.17(1)(a)(iii); r 17(1)(a)(iii)
6. Ibid, r 4.17; r 17
7. John Spencer and Rhona Flin *The Evidence of Children* (Blackstone Press, 1991) (a very readable and informed book on the law and psychology of children's evidence) and Richard May *Criminal Evidence* (Sweet & Maxwell, 1990) (a useful textbook on the law of evidence in criminal cases)
8. The Children (Admissibility of Hearsay Evidence) Order 1991, SI 1991/1115
9. *Pigot Committee Report* (Home Office, 1989); Criminal Justice Act 1991, ss 52–55
10. *Memorandum of Good Practice on Video-recorded Interviews with Child Witnesses for Criminal Proceedings* (HMSO, 1992)

Chapter 14

EXPERT EVIDENCE

Before an expert witness is called to give oral evidence in court, his written report should have been sent to the court and the other parties in the case. Usually, the instructing solicitor arranges a conference with the barrister or solicitor representing the client [1].

Experts to be called by opposing parties should have an opportunity to confer with each other, exchanging views. It is often productive to discuss points at issue before a case, clarifying differences of opinion and ensuring that any differences do not result from a failure to fully inform the experts.

In preparing reports, it is useful to record in logical order: sources; a summary of relevant facts; information elicited; conclusions drawn; the reasoning and experiential basis upon which those conclusions are reached, and research and other work cited.

Many expert reports are accepted without oral evidence. When a witness is asked to come to court, it is vital to make a good impression, and not to lose the impact of a competent report by inept evidence. David Carson, in his excellent book for expert witnesses [2], explains how to enhance self-presentation in court, and how to maintain attention coupled with respect for the evidence given. With humour, he also suggests some very effective ways of dealing with cross-examination. Gee and Mason [3] give helpful information on courtroom techniques, including in their text some specific medical situations.

BE PREPARED

Experienced advocates agree that their most effective work is done outside court. Expert evidence is the same. The preparation which goes into writing a report pays dividends in court.

Before going to the court, read through all notes, diagrams, charts, and research which are mentioned in the report, or which may be necessary in explaining opinions or conclusions. Make sure that in the file, there are copies of everything to which reference is required. If the case is complex, have a chronology. Ensure that the names of the parties are clearly memorised. It is inefficient not to include the names of those people who have instructed your report, or the names of the other parties.

Files should be arranged so that individual papers required in court can be found and extracted without fuss. If an advocate asks to look at a particular item, you should be able to have it to hand quickly. Make sure you know where everything is in the file.

Experts are often allowed to sit in on the case, and it can be productive to hear the other evidence given, perhaps for the first time. However, there could be a long wait outside the courtroom, in a draughty waiting area, without easy access to a canteen or telephone. It is therefore advisable to take something with you to pass the time while waiting to be called. Dress should be appropriate to a professional image.

WHERE TO GO ON ARRIVAL AT COURT

The family proceedings court is usually separate from the criminal section of the magistrates' court. Ushers (usually in black gowns, clutching clipboards) will sign in the advocates and show witnesses to the appropriate courtroom. High Courts and county courts similarly have ushers. They are great sources of information, and are there to help. Always report in to an usher and get help to find the right courtroom. If you arrive late, this is especially important. Many a witness has waited outside the wrong court unannounced while the case is held up waiting for them. The court's permission has to be sought before a witness sits in on a case. Otherwise, a witness has to wait outside the court until called. If taking a break, always tell the usher where you are so that if necessary, he or she can explain to the court your absence, or come to find you.

Never leave papers and files unattended outside a court. If the case is adjourned over lunch or overnight, ensure that the room will be locked if papers are to be left there. It is generally preferable to keep your papers with you.

IN THE WITNESS BOX

Oath or Affirmation?

Decide, before entering court, whether you want to take the oath or affirm. The oath is still more frequently chosen but the court will respect either choice. The court will not be impressed, however, if you dither over your decision. Read the words on the card carefully, even if you know them well. Trying to memorise them, then tripping over the words will not enhance your professional image.

What to call Magistrates and Judges

In the family proceedings court, magistrates may be called 'sir' or 'madam', addressing your evidence to the chairperson in the middle. Magistrates may also be called 'your worship' but this is becoming less frequently used.

County court and crown court judges are called 'your honour' whether they are male or female.

High Court judges, and all judges at the central criminal court (the Old Bailey) are 'my lord' or 'my lady'.

Subtleties and Power Games

Courtroom tactics involve power games. It is important not to become involved in these. There are many subtle put-downs which advocates may engage in. Fortunately, these usually by-pass non-lawyers. Some, however, are useful to know. 'I hear what you say' means 'I heard what you said, but I don't believe or accept it'; 'With respect' implies the opposite; and 'Perhaps you would just like to refer again to your notes?' is either to put you off your guard or is a warning that something important has been omitted, or there is an error somewhere.

A tactic you can employ yourself if you are being pressurised is to ask the court for time to consult your notes. If you need time to consult your notes, ask for it. For example, 'Would the court please grant me a moment to consult my notes?'. Do not allow yourself to be rushed. Your role as an expert witness is to give clear, accurate evidence to the court. If you are rushed or nervous you may be less able to do this well.

If you need to use the lavatory, the traditional request is 'May I ask for a short adjournment for personal reasons, please?' Most courts will understand and grant it. If pressed, state the reason without embarrassment.

Most courts will offer a witness the chance to sit down. If this is not offered, and illness or infirmity make sitting necessary, do not hesitate to ask. Courts will grant such requests if they are clearly made.

Giving Evidence

When you give your evidence, be concise, and avoid jargon or technicalities wherever possible. If technical terms are vital, explain their meaning clearly, but not in a patronising way. Lack of knowledge on the part of the court, jury, or lawyers is not indicative of lack of intelligence! Look politely at the person asking the question, then, turn to the magistrates or judge when answering. Carson [4] points out the advantages of the thinking time so gained, and also the effect of looking away from an advocate when answering. Interruptions from an advocate are a typical cross-examination technique. They may irritate you but take advantage of them to give yourself time to keep calm, and finish giving your evidence before tackling the interruption. Even better, turn briefly back to the advocate, saying something like: 'Please let me finish, then I will answer your next question' and turn deliberately back to the magistrates or judge to complete whatever you were saying.

Don't be led into saying more than you want or need to say, or feel compelled to stop what you were saying to answer an advocate who has interrupted your evidence.

Stages in Giving Evidence

The first stage in giving evidence is examination in chief. The party calling the witness asks the first questions to elicit the facts required. This is followed by cross-examination – questions from the other parties or their advocates – then re-examination by the instructing party to tie up loose ends raised in the evidence. Finally, there are questions from the court, the judge or magistrates. The court will then either release the witness, who is free to leave the court, or will ask the witness to remain available in case he or she is needed again. Do not leave the court unless you are released. It is quite acceptable to ask the court before leaving the witness box 'May I be released now please?', if the advocate calling you has not done so.

Who can an Expert Witness Speak to Outside Court?

Nobody owns a witness or his evidence. Sometimes there can be difficulties for an inexperienced witness who is engaged in conversation outside the courtroom by a legal representative and may be tackled on a controversial point, then later finds that unguarded remarks are quoted back at him in court. Barristers, traditionally, were not allowed to speak to witnesses directly (even their own witnesses), but had to converse through, or in the presence of, their instructing solicitor. This is gradually relaxing, but do not feel snubbed if this happens. It is advisable, if approached by anyone to discuss a case outside court, to politely insist that your instructing solicitor be present. In children cases, the spirit of the Act encourages full and frank disclosure of all facts relevant to the interests of the child, so all discussion should be encouraged, particularly between experts.

PAYMENT

The fees payable for court reports and for court attendance are negotiable. If the client for whom the expert witness is called is legally aided, then the Legal Aid Board will want to authorise fees in advance of the case. It helps if the witness can give the person calling witnesses an estimate of the cost before undertaking the work, and ensuring that there is a contract for the service to be provided, usually by exchange of letters. Write to confirm any agreed terms, if they are negotiated by telephone. Some solicitors pay immediately on completion of the case, others wait for their bill to be paid before paying witnesses. Clarify this as part of the negotiations on accepting instructions. There are guidelines as to fees for criminal cases agreed by the British Medical Association and the Crown Prosecution Service; these vary from time to time. For civil cases, there are no fixed guidelines. It is important to settle fees beforehand, and if necessary, the solicitor will obtain authorisation from the Legal Aid Board or the client for the expenditure.

Fees may be charged at an hourly rate or a fixed fee for preparation of reports. Travelling expenses may also be claimed, in mileage or fares. Fees for practitioners' attendance at court may be charged on an hourly basis, or by the half or full day, as appropriate.

Many lawyers say that it helps billing if witnesses render their fee notes as soon as possible after the conclusion of a case. A note of the time spent in preparation, report writing and attendance at court can be vital in justifying the expenditure.

INTER-DISCIPLINARY COMMUNICATION

The organisations listed below aim to encourage inter-disciplinary communication and best forensic practice. They also provide the opportunity to attend meetings, seminars and conferences, and publish journals and other material which may be of interest to the practitioner.

The Forensic Science Society
Clarke House
18a Mount Parade
Harrogate
North Yorkshire HG1 1BX
(This society also publishes a list of independent consultants in various geographical areas and fields of expertise.)

The Medico-Legal Society
Hon Legal Secretary: Miss Pygott
Beaufort House
15 St Botolph Street
London EC3A 7NJ

British Academy of Forensic Sciences
Secretariat
Department of Anaesthesia
The Royal London Hospital
Turner Street
London E1 2AD

Also of interest, a new international journal:
Expert Evidence
SLE Publications Ltd
77 Birdham Road
Chichester
West Sussex PO20 7BR

REFERENCES

1. For details about reports, preparation and service, see Chapter 13
2. D Carson *Professionals and the Courts* (Venture Press, 1990)
3. D J Gee and J K Mason *The Courts and the Doctor* (Oxford Medical Publications, 1990)
4. Carson, op. cit.

GLOSSARY

The Children Act 1989 provides, in s 105, the interpretation of many specific terms used. Other sections of the Act also give definitions, or refer to other enactments. Those relevant are also included here. In the text we have used some terms of our own; these, too, are included. To avoid confusion, we have indicated with an asterisk those terms which are not formally defined by legislation. The wording of the Act, wherever cited below, is indicated by quotation marks.

adoption agency   'a body which may be referred to as an adoption agency by virtue of section 1 of the Adoption Act 1976' (includes a local authority).

authorised person   in relation to care and supervision proceedings, means a person (other than a local authority) authorised by order of the Secretary of State to bring care or supervision proceedings under s 31 of the Act, including any officer of a body so authorised. In the Act there are other persons authorised to carry out specified functions, ie to inspect premises used for private fostering.

bank holiday   'a day which is a bank holiday under the Banking and Financial Dealings Act 1971' (includes all the usual bank holidays in the UK).

care order   an order made under s 31(1)(a), (placement
                             of a child in the care of a local authority)
                             including an order made under s 38 (an
                             interim order placing a child in the care of a
                             local authority); and 'includes any order
                             which is deemed by any enactment to be, or
                             to have the effect of, a care order for the
                             purposes of this Act; and any reference to a
                             child who is in the care of an authority is a
                             reference to a child who is in their care by
                             virtue of a care order'.

child   'a person under the age of eighteen'.

child in care   a child in the care of a local authority
                             pursuant to an order made or deemed to be
                             made under s 31(1)(a) or an interim order
                             under s 38 of the Act.

child in need   'a child shall be taken to be in need if –

                             (a) he is unlikely to achieve or maintain, or
                                 to have the opportunity of achieving or
                                 maintaining, a reasonable standard of
                                 health or development without the
                                 provision for him of services by a local
                                 authority;
                             (b) his health or development is likely to be
                                 significantly impaired, or further
                                 impaired, without the provision for him
                                 of such services; or
                             (c) he is disabled,' s 17(10).

                             Note: There is a duty under s 17(1) on every
                             local authority to safeguard and promote the
                             welfare of children in need within their area;
                             and so far as is consistent with that duty, to
                             promote the upbringing of those children by
                             their families by provision of a range of
                             services appropriate to those children's
                             needs.

child of the family 'in relation to the parties to a marriage, means –

(a) a child of both of those parties;
(b) any other child, not being a child who is placed with those parties as foster parents by a local authority or voluntary organisation, who has been treated by both of those parties as a child of their family;', s 105(1)

child looked after by a local authority is a child who is in the care of a local authority by virtue of a care order, or provided with accommodation by a local authority.

child provided with accommodation by a local authority is a child who is provided with accommodation by a local authority in the exercise of its functions, particularly those under the Act, which stand referred to their social services committee under the Local Authorities Social Services Act 1970 (includes children in what was previously called voluntary care).

children's home is defined in s 63 as a home that provides, or usually provides, or is intended to provide care and accommodation wholly or mainly for more than three children at any one time. Obviously, many homes contain three or more children, and the section lists several exceptions, including homes of parents, relatives, or those with parental responsibility for the child in question.

community home is defined in s 53(3); and may be a home:

'(a) provided, managed, equipped and maintained by a local authority; or
(b) provided by a voluntary organisation but in respect of which a local authority and the organisation –

(i) propose that, in accordance with an instrument of management, the management, equipment and maintenance of the home shall be the responsibility of the local authority; or

(ii) so propose that the management, equipment and maintenance of the home shall be the responsibility of the voluntary organisation.'

contact order

'"a contact order" means an order requiring the person with whom a child lives, or is to live, to allow the child to visit or stay with the person named in the order, or for that person and the child otherwise to have contact with each other;', s 8(1).

the court

means the High Court, county court or a magistrates' court, s 92(7). The High Court and county court have a Family Division and the magistrates have a Family Proceedings Court.

development

'means physical, intellectual, emotional, social or behavioural development', s 17(11).

disabled

in relation to a child, 'a child is disabled if he is blind, deaf or dumb or suffers from mental disorder of any kind or is substantially and permanently handicapped by illness, injury or congenital deformity or such other disability as may be prescribed', s 17(11).

district health authority

remains as defined in the National Health Service Act 1977 'The health authority for a district, whether or not the name incorporates the word "district"'.

domestic premises

any premises (including any vehicle) used wholly or mainly as a private dwelling.

**education
supervision order**

means an order under s 36(1) of the Act, putting the child with respect to whom the order is made under the supervision of a designated local education authority.

**emergency
protection order**

an order made under s 44(4) of the Act:

'(a) operates as a direction to any person who is in a position to do so to comply with any request to produce the child . . .
(b) authorises –
  (i) the removal of the child at any time to accommodation provided by or on behalf of the applicant and his [the child] being kept there; or
  (ii) the prevention of the child's removal from any hospital, or other place, in which he was being accommodated immediately before the making of the order; and
(c) gives the applicant parental responsibility for the child.'

**family assistance
order**

an order made under s 16 of the Act appointing a probation officer or an officer of the local authority to advise assist and befriend a named person for a period of six months or less. Named persons may include parents, guardians, those with whom the child lives, or the child himself.

family proceedings

defined in s 8(3) and (4) as any proceedings:

'(a) under the inherent jurisdiction of the High Court in relation to children;', s 8(3)

'(a) Parts I, II and IV of this Act;
(b) the Matrimonial Causes Act 1973;
(c) the Domestic Violence and Matrimonial Proceedings Act 1976;
(d) the Adoption Act 1976;

(e) the Domestic Proceedings and
     Magistrates' Courts Act 1978;
(f) sections 1 and 9 of the Matrimonial
     Homes Act 1983;
(g) Part III of the Matrimonial and Family
     Proceedings Act 1984,' s 8(4)
(See Figure 1.3 above *Legal Procedures to
Protect Children.*)

**family proceedings
court**

is the part of the magistrates' court which
deals with Children Act cases and other
family matters.

harm

defined in s 31(9) means ill-treatment or the
impairment of health or development, and
where the question of whether the harm is
significant or not turns on the child's health
and development, the child's health or
development shall be compared with that
which could be reasonably expected of a
similar child.

health

defined in s 17(11) to include physical or
mental health.

health authority

means any district health authority and any
special health authority established under the
National Health Service Act 1977.

**health service
hospital**

a hospital vested in the Secretary of State
under the National Health Service Act 1977.

hospital

any health service hospital, and
accommodation provided by the local
authority and used as a hospital. It does not
include special hospitals, which are those for
people detained under the Mental Health Act
1983, providing secure hospital
accommodation.

ill-treatment

defined in s 31(9) and includes sexual abuse
and forms of ill-treatment which are not
physical.

independent school	any school offering full-time education for five or more pupils of compulsory school age not being a school maintained by a local education authority.
local authority	means a council of a county, a metropolitan district, a London borough, or the Common Council of the City of London; in Scotland, it means a local authority under the Social Work (Scotland) Act 1968, s 12.
local authority foster parent	means any person with whom a child has been placed by a local authority under s 23(2)(a) of the Act. The local authority foster parent may be a family; a relative of the child; or any other suitable person.
local education authority	means in relation to any area for which a joint education board is constituted as a local education authority under Part 1, Sch 1, of the Education Act 1944, the board; or the council of the county; or the council of the county borough.
local housing authority	is defined in the Housing Act 1944 as the district council; London borough council; Common council of the City of London; or council of the Isles of Scilly.
mental nursing home	defined in the Registered Homes Act 1984 as 'any premises used . . . for the reception of and provision of nursing or other medical treatment . . . for one or more mentally disordered patients, whether exclusively or in common with other persons'.
*non-parent with parental responsibility	a person who is not a natural parent of a child, but who has parental responsibility for the child

nursing home	as defined in the Registered Homes Act 1984 any premises used or intended to be used for reception or nursing for sickness, injury or infirmity; and for pregnant women or childbirth; or certain specified medical procedures, including termination of pregnancies.
*parent	the natural mother or father of a child, whether or not they are married to each other at the time of the birth or of conception.
parental responsibility	defined in s 3 as 'all the rights, duties, powers, responsibilities and authority which by law a parent of a child has in relation to the child and his property'.
parental responsibility agreement	defined in s 4(1). A formal agreement between the father and mother of a child providing for the father to have parental responsibility for the child (a father married to the mother of their child at or after the child's birth will automatically have parental responsibility for that child, but an unmarried father will not). There is a prescribed form and registration procedure for these agreements. See Chapter 2 for details.
*parent with parental responsibility	a parent who has, or has acquired parental responsibility for a child. This term will *not* include a natural father of a child if he has not acquired parental responsibility under the Act, nor will it include a step-parent unless he or she has formally acquired parental responsibility. See Chapter 2.
prescribed	means prescribed by regulations under the Act.

privately fostered child

defined in s 66 'to foster a child privately' means looking after a child under the age of 16 (or if disabled, 18), caring and providing accommodation for him or her; by someone who is not the child's parent, relative, or who has parental responsibility for the child.

prohibited steps order

defined in s 8 means an order that no step that could be taken by a parent in meeting his or her parental responsibility for a child, and that is of a kind specified in the order, shall be taken by any person without the consent of the court.

protected child

is a child protected under the Adoption Act 1976, ie a child who is living with the applicant to adopt the child, who has given notice to the local authority of his or her intention to apply to adopt. The child is subject to the supervision of the local authority during the period of protection, which continues until one of a number of specified circumstances occur.

residence order

defined in s 8 as an order settling the arrangements to be made as to the person with whom a child is to live.

residential care home

defined in s 1 of the Registered Homes Act 1984. Basically, an establishment where four or more people in need of personal care because of old age, disablement, past or present dependence on alcohol or drugs, or mental disorder, must be registered as a residential care home, with the result that conditions may be imposed as to its use.

registered children's home

defined in s 63 as a home, registered under the Act, which provides (or usually provides or is intended to provide) care and accommodation wholly or mainly for more than three children, who are not siblings with respect to each other, at any one time. Section 63 provides a number of exceptions to the category of children's homes.

registered pupil

in relation to a school, a pupil registered at that school.

relative

in relation to a child means a grandparent, brother, sister, uncle or aunt (whether of the full blood or of the half blood or by affinity) or step-parent.

responsible person

defined in Sch 3, Part I, para 1 in relation to a supervised child means

'(a) any person who has parental responsibility for the child; and
(b) any other person with whom the child is living'.

service

in relation to any provision made under Part III of the Act (local authority support for children and families) means any facility.

*signed

in relation to any person includes the making of his or her mark. For some purposes, such as the appointment of a guardian, the document may be signed by another at the direction of the appointer and witnessed by two people.

special educational needs

these arise when there is a learning difficulty that calls for special educational provision to be made. The Education Act 1981, s 1(1), sets out the meaning of 'learning difficulty'.

special health authority	defined in the National Health Service Act 1977 as a special body established to perform functions on behalf of an area or district health authority, or Family Practitioner Committee (now the FHSA).
specific issue order	defined in s 8(1) as an order giving directions for the purpose of determining a specific issue that has arisen, or that may arise, in connection with any aspect of parental responsibility for a child.
supervision order	means an order under s 31(1)(b) and (except where express provision to the contrary is made), includes an interim supervision order made under s 38.
supervised child and **supervisor**	in relation to a supervision order or an education supervision order, mean respectively the child who is (or is to be) under supervision and the person under whose supervision he or she is (or is to be) by virtue of the order.
upbringing	in relation to any child includes the care of the child but not his or her maintenance.
voluntary home	means any home or other institution providing care and accommodation for children which is carried on by a voluntary organisation, with certain exceptions set out in s 60 of the Act.
voluntary organisation	means a body (other than a public or local authority) whose activities are not carried on for profit.

This glossary (with slight amendments for the purposes of this book) is reproduced with kind permission of Longman from *The Children Act 1989 – A Practical Guide* by Linda Feldman and Barbara Mitchels.

APPENDIX 1

CONFIDENTIALITY AND DISCLOSURE OF MEDICAL INFORMATION

Disclosure of information held by health professionals about their patients is frequently requested for litigation or other purposes. Below is a brief summary of the current statutory provisions controlling the disclosure of information, as influenced by the Children Act 1989.

Data Protection Act 1984

Protects information held on computer. Section 21 allows patients access to health records kept on computer, with exemptions specified in the **Data Protection Act (Subject Access Modification) (Health) Order 1987, SI 1987/1903**. Also refer to the **Data Protection Act (Subject Access Modification) (Social Work) Order 1987, SI 1987/1904**.

If information is requested about a child, it is suggested that the appropriate person to seek that information is a person with parental responsibility for that child, and that if the child is 16 years of age or is *Gillick* competent, ie of sufficient maturity and understanding to make his own medical decisions, then his instructions regarding disclosure should be solicited and respected.

Access to Personal Files Act 1987 and The Access to Personal Files (Social Services) Regulations 1989, SI 1989/206

Gives a right of access by individuals to those records about them which are not stored on a computer. It applies to local authority records relating to their housing and social services functions. Some social services records will contain medical information provided by health professionals about individuals. There are safeguards in this Act against the disclosure of particular information which may not be in that individual's best interests. Each case must be considered on its own merits. Solicitors or others requiring information on behalf of a client would expect to produce a written consent from their client for that request. See also **Local Authority Circular LAC (89)2**. If information is requested about a child, the appropriate applicant is a person with parental responsibility for that child, or a solicitor instructed by the child if he is of sufficient understanding, or by a guardian ad litem on the child's behalf.

The guardian ad litem appointed by the court in a Children Act case has a separate statutory right of access to social services records given by the **Children Act 1989, s 42**.

Access to Health Records Act 1990

This Act applies to all records relating to physical or mental health of an identifiable individual which have been made by a health professional in connection with the care of that individual and treatment. It does not include computerised records which are already covered by the Data Protection Act 1984.

The term 'health professional' is defined in s 2 of the Act. Access to records may be sought by those specified in s 3 of the Act including: the patient in writing, or a person with parental responsibility for a child patient, or in Scotland, the parent or guardian of a pupil.

The applicant may inspect the record or extracts from it, and request a copy, together with an explanation of terms which would otherwise be unintelligible.

Where the patient is a child, the health professional must be satisfied that either:

- they understand the nature of the application if they want access themselves or have authorised it; or
- if the applicant has parental responsibility for the child, the health practitioner must be satisfied that the child agrees, or is incapable of agreeing and that the access requested is in the child's best interests (s 4).

Access may be wholly or partly refused on grounds specified in the Act, which include circumstances where the disclosure would cause serious harm to the physical or mental health of the patient or another individual. Access may also be denied where it would lead to disclosure of the identity of another individual who has provided information, unless that individual consents or is another health professional involved in the care of the patient.

Clearly, in cases where there is an investigation of child abuse, access to records may become an important issue. It is here that inter-agency co-operation becomes vital. See Chapter 12 for further discussion. Also, see *Working Together Under the Children Act 1989 (HMSO 1992)* which provides useful guidance, and the following quotation from the Annual Report 1987 of the General Medical Council which gives this clear advice on the matter of confidentiality and disclosure of information in cases of child abuse. It still stands.

'The Council's published guidance on professional confidence states that doctors may disclose confidential information to the police who are investigating a grave or very serious crime, provided always that they are prepared to justify their actions if called upon to do so. However, a specialist in child psychiatry recently drew to the Council's attention that its guidance does not specifically address the question of whether a doctor may properly initiate action in a case of this kind, as opposed to responding to a request. Both the British Medical Association and the medical defence societies have expressed the view that in such circumstances the interests of the child are paramount and that those interests may well override the general rule of professional confidence. On the recommendation of the Standards Committee, the Council in November 1987 expressed the view that, if a doctor has reason for believing that a child is being physically or sexually abused, not only is it permissible for the doctor to disclose information to a third party but it is a duty of the doctor to do so.'

The General Medical Council advised in 1991 that where a doctor judges that a child patient does not have sufficient understanding to give a valid consent

'he may decide to disclose the information learned from the consultation, but if he does so, he should inform the patient accordingly, and his judgment concerning disclosure must always reflect both the patient's best medical interests and the trust that the patient places in the doctor.'

Also of interest is the Memorandum on Child Abuse and Confidentiality from the Joint Co-ordinating Committee of the UK Medical Defence organisations quoted in 'Diagnosis of Child Sexual Abuse: Guidance for Doctors (Standing Medical Advisory Committee DHSS 1988).

The local Area Child Protection Committee guidelines are now being rewritten to take into account the provisions of the Children Act, and will be available for practitioners' reference.

APPENDIX 2

ANNOTATED EXTRACTS FROM THE CURRENT EDITION OF A GUIDE TO CONSENT FOR EXAMINATION AND TREATMENT (NHS MANAGEMENT EXECUTIVE)

Advising the Patient

1. Where a choice of treatment might reasonably be offered the health professional may always advise the patient of his or her recommendations together with reasons for selecting a particular course of action. Normally enough information must be given to ensure that the patient understands the nature, consequences and any substantial risks of the treatment proposed so that they are able to take a decision based on that information. Though it should be assumed that most patients will wish to be well informed, account should be taken of those who may find this distressing.

2. The patient's ability to appreciate the significance of the information should be assessed. For example with patients who:
   i.   may be shocked, distressed or in pain;
   ii. have difficulty in understanding English or Welsh;
   iii. have impaired sight, or hearing or speech;
   iv. are suffering from mental disability but who nevertheless have the capacity to give consent to the proposed procedure.

3. Occasionally and subject to the agreement of the patient, and where circumstances permit, it may help if a close family member or a friend can be present at the discussion when consent is sought. If this is not possible another member of the staff may be able to assist the patient in understanding. Where there are language problems, it is important an interpreter be sought whenever possible.

4. A doctor will have to exercise his or her professional skill and judgement in deciding what risks the patient should be warned of and the terms in which the warning should be given. However, a

doctor has a duty to warn patients of substantial or unusual risk inherent in any proposed treatment. This is especially so with surgery but may apply to other procedures including drug therapy and radiation treatment. Guidance on the amount of information and warnings of risk to be given to patients can be found in the judgment of the House of Lords in the case of *Sidaway v Gov of Bethlem Royal Hospital* [1985] AC 87.

[*Note.* See p 144 below]

Obtaining Consent

5. Consent to treatment may be implied or expressed. In many cases patients do not explicitly give express consent but their agreement may be implied by compliant actions, eg by offering an arm for the taking of a blood sample. Express consent is given when patients confirm their agreement to a procedure or treatment in clear and explicit terms, whether orally or in writing.

6. Oral consent may be sufficient for the vast majority of contacts with patients by doctors and nurses and other health professionals. Written consent should be obtained for any procedure or treatment carrying any substantial risk or substantial side-effect. If the patient is capable, written consent should always be obtained for general anaesthesia, surgery, certain forms of drug therapy, eg cytotoxic therapy and therapy involving the use of ionising radiation. Oral or written consent should be recorded in the patient's notes with relevant details of the health professional's explanation. Where written consent is obtained it should be incorporated into the notes.

7. *Standard consent form.* The main purpose of written consent is to provide documentary evidence that an explanation of the proposed procedure or treatment was given and that consent was sought and obtained. The model consent forms set out the requirements for obtaining valid consent to treatment in terms that will be readily understood by the patient. In the majority of cases these forms will be used by registered medical or dental staff but there may be occasions when other health professionals will wish to record formally that consent has been obtained for a particular procedure. A separate form is available for their use.

8. It should be noted that the purpose of obtaining a signature on the consent form is not an end in itself. The most important element of a

consent procedure is the duty to ensure that patients understand the nature and purpose of the proposed treatment. Where a patient has not been given appropriate information then consent may not always have been obtained despite the signature on the form.

9. Consent given for one procedure or episode of treatment does not give any automatic right to undertake any other procedure. A doctor may, however, undertake further treatment if the circumstances are such that a patient's consent cannot reasonably be requested and provided the treatment is immediately necessary and the patient has not previously indicated that the further treatment would be unacceptable.

Special Circumstances

Treatment of Children and Young People

[*Editorial note*: This was written prior to implementation of the Children Act 1989 and references to 'parent' and 'parental consent' should now imply a parent with parental responsibility or other person with parental responsibility for the child, or the consent of such a person. For further discussion, see Chapters 3 and 10.]

10. *Children under the age of 16 years.* Where a child under the age of 16 achieves a sufficient understanding of what is proposed, that child may consent to a doctor or other health professional making an examination and giving treatment. The doctor or health professional must be satisfied that any such child has sufficient understanding of what is involved in the treatment that is proposed. A full note should be made of the factors taken into account by the doctor in making his or her assessment of the child's capacity to give a valid consent. In the majority of cases children will be accompanied by their parents during consultations. Where, exceptionally, a child is seen alone, efforts should be made to persuade the child that his or her parents should be informed except in circumstances where it is clearly not in the child's best interests to do so. [Parental consent] should be obtained where a child does not have sufficient understanding and is under age 16 except in an emergency where there is not time to obtain it.

11. *Young people over the age of 16 years.* The effect of s 8 of the Family Law Reform Act 1969 is that the consent of a young person who has

attained 16 years to any surgical, medical or dental treatment is sufficient in itself and it is not necessary to obtain a separate consent from the [parent] or guardian. In cases where a child is over age 16 but is not competent to give a valid consent, then the consent of a [parent] or guardian must be sought. However, such power only extends until that child is 18.

12. *Refusal of [parental consent] to urgent or life-saving treatment.* Where time permits, court action may be taken so that consent may be obtained from a judge. Otherwise hospital authorities should rely on the clinical judgement of the doctors, normally the consultants, concerned after a full discussion between the doctor and the parents. In such a case the doctor should obtain a written supporting opinion from a medical colleague that the patient's life is in danger if the treatment is withheld and should discuss the need to treat with the parents or guardian in the presence of a witness. The doctor should record the discussion in the clinical notes and ask the witness to countersign the record. In these circumstances and where practicable the doctor may wish to consult his or her defence organisation. If he or she has followed the procedure set out above and has then acted in the best interests of the patient and with due professional competence and according to their own professional conscience, they are unlikely to be criticised by a court or by their professional body.

Adult or Competent Young Person Refusing Treatment

13. Some adult patients will wish to refuse some parts of their treatment. This will include those whose religious beliefs prevent them accepting a blood transfusion. Whatever the reason for the refusal such patients should receive a detailed explanation of the nature of their illness and the need for the treatment or transfusion proposed. They should also be warned in clear terms that the doctor may properly decline to modify the procedure and of the possible consequences if the procedure is not carried out. If the patient then refuses to agree, and he or she is competent, the refusal must be respected. The doctor should record this in the clinical notes and where possible have it witnessed.

[*Editorial note*: see the recent cases of *Re E*, *Re R* and *Re J* discussed in Chapter 10, in particular *Re J* at p 65 and the *Gillick* case, together with *Re E* and *Re R* at pp 66–69, and pp 71–73.]

Teaching on Patients

14. Detailed guidance about medical students in hospitals is the subject of a separate circular to be issued shortly. It should not be assumed, especially in a teaching hospital, that a patient is available for teaching purposes or for practical experience by clinical, medical or dental or other staff under training.

Examination or Treatment without the patient's consent

15. The following are examples of occasions when examination or treatment may proceed without obtaining the patient's consent:
    i. For life-saving procedures where the patient is unconscious and cannot indicate his or her wishes.
    ii. Where there is a statutory power requiring the examination of a patient, for example, under the Public Health (Control of Disease) Act 1984. However an explanation should be offered and the patient's co-operation should nevertheless be sought.
    iii. In certain cases where a minor is a ward of court and the court decides that a specific treatment is in the child's best interests.
    iv. Treatment for mental disorder of a patient liable to be detained in hospital under the Mental Health Act 1983.
    v. Treatment for physical disorder where the patient is incapable of giving consent by reason of mental disorder, and the treatment is in the patient's best interest.

FAMILY LAW REFORM ACT 1969 S 8

Consent by Person Over 16 to Surgical, Medical and Dental Treatment

1. The consent of a minor who has attained the age of sixteen years to any surgical, medical or dental treatment which, in the absence of consent, would constitute a trespass to his person, shall be as effective as it would be if he were of full age; and where a minor has by virtue of this section given an effective consent to any treatment it shall not be necessary to obtain any consent for it from his parent or guardian.
2. In this section 'surgical, medical or dental treatment' includes any procedure undertaken for the purpose of diagnosis, and this section

applies to any procedure (including, in particular, the administration of an anaesthetic) which is ancillary to any treatment as it applies to that treatment.

3. Nothing in this section shall be construed as making ineffective any consent which would have been effective if this section had not been enacted.

EXAMPLES OF TREATMENTS WHICH HAVE RAISED CONCERN

Maternity Services

1. Principles of consent are the same in maternity services as in other areas of medicine. It is important that the proposed care is discussed with the woman, preferably in the early antenatal period, when any special wishes she expresses should be recorded in the notes, but of course the patient may change her mind about these issues at any stage, including during labour.

2. Decisions may have to be taken swiftly at a time when the woman's ability to give consent is impaired, eg as a result of medication, including analgesics. If the safety of the woman or child is at stake the obstetrician or midwife should take any reasonable action that is necessary. If, in the judgment of the relevant health professional, the woman is temporarily unable to make a decision, it may be advisable for the position to be explained to her husband or partner if available, but his consent (or withholding of consent) cannot legally override the clinical judgment of the health professional, as guided by the previously expressed wishes of the patient herself.

Breast Cancer

3. The usual principles of explaining proposed treatment and obtaining the patient's consent should be followed in treating cases of breast cancer. Breast cancer does not normally require emergency treatment. The patient needs reassurance that a mastectomy will not be performed without her consent, and that unless she has indicated otherwise the need for any further surgery will be fully discussed with her in the light of biopsy and other results. This is a particular case of the principle [set out in point 9, p 137] that consent to an initial treatment or investigation does not imply consent to further treatment.

Tissue and Organ Donation – Risk of Transmitted Infection

4. Where tissues or organs are to be transplanted, the recipient should be informed at the time when consent to operation is obtained of the small, but unavoidable risk of the transplant being infected. Further guidance is available in a CMO letter, *HIV Infection, Tissue Banks and Organ Donation* (PL/CMO/92).

CONSENT BY PATIENTS SUFFERING FROM MENTAL DISORDER

1. Consent to treatment must be given freely and without coercion and be based on information about the nature, purpose and likely effects of treatment presented in a way that it is understandable by the patient. The capacity of the person to understand the information given will depend on their intellectual state, the nature of their mental disorder, and any variability over time of their mental state. The ability of mentally disordered people to make and communicate decisions may similarly vary from time to time.
2. The presence of mental disorder does not by itself imply incapacity, nor does detention under the Mental Health Act. Each patient's capability for giving consent, has to be judged individually in the light of the nature of the decision required and the mental state of the patient at the time.

Mental Health Legislation – Treatment for Mental Disorders

3. The Mental Health Act 1983 took a major step forward in providing for mentally disordered people, detained in hospital under the powers of the Act, to be given treatment for *mental disorder*, without their consent where they are incapable of giving consent. Certain procedures and safeguards are laid down in relation to specific groups of treatment, including the need for multidisciplinary discussion and the agreement of doctors appointed to give a second opinion.

Mental Incapacity and Treatment for Physical Conditions

4. The Mental Health Act 1983 does not contain provisions to enable treatment of *physical disorders* without consent either for detained

patients or those people who may be suffering from mental disorder but who are not detained under the Mental Health Act.

The administration of treatment for physical conditions to people incapable of giving consent and making their own treatment decisions is a matter of concern to all involved in the care of such people, whether they are detained in hospital or in hospital but non-detained, in residential care or in the community.

The House of Lords' Decision in *In Re F* [1989] 2 WLR 1025; [1989] 2 All ER 525

5. This decision helped to clarify the common law in relation to general medical and surgical treatment of people who lack the capacity to give consent. No one may give consent on behalf of an adult but the substantive law is that a proposed operation or treatment is lawful if it is in the best interests of the patient and unlawful if it is not. Guidance given in that case is set out below:

i.   In considering the lawfulness of medical and surgical treatment given to a patient who for any reason, temporary or permanent, lacks the capacity to give or to communicate consent to treatment, it was stated to be axiomatic that treatment that is necessary to preserve the life, health or well-being of the patient may lawfully be given without consent.

ii. The standard of care required of the doctor concerned in all cases is laid down in *Bolam v Friern Hospital Management Committee* [1957] 1 WLR 582, namely, that he or she must act in accordance with a responsible body of relevant professional opinion.

iii. In many cases, it will not only be lawful for doctors, on the ground of necessity to operate or give other medical treatment to adult patients disabled from giving their consent, it will also be their common law duty to do so.

iv. In the case of the mentally disordered, when the state is permanent or semi-permanent, action properly taken, may well transcend such matters as surgical operation or substantial medical treatment and may extend to include such (humdrum) matters as routine medical and dental treatment and even simple care such as dressing and undressing and putting to bed.

v.   In practice, a decision may involve others besides the doctor. It must surely be good practice to consult relatives and others who are concerned with the care of the patient. Sometimes, of course, consultation with a specialist or specialists will be required; and in others, especially where the decision involves more than a purely medical opinion, an inter-disciplinary team will in practice participate in the decision.

Documentation

6. Proposals for treatment should as a matter of good practice, be discussed with the multidisciplinary team and where necessary other doctors and, with the consent of the patient where this is possible, with their nearest relative or friend. The decisions taken should be documented in the clinical case notes. In cases involving anaesthesia, and surgery, or where the treatment carries substantial or unusual risk it would also be advisable for documentation to record that the patient is incapable of giving consent to treatment and that the doctor in charge of the patient's treatment is of the opinion that the treatment proposed should be given and that it is in the patient's best interests. A model form is suggested to register medical opinion – where a patient is incapable of giving consent.

Sterilisation

7. In *Re F* it was said that special features applied in the case of an operation for sterilisation. Having regard to those matters, it was stated to be highly desirable as a matter of good practice to involve the court in the decision to operate. In practice an application should be made to a court whenever it is proposed to perform such an operation. The procedure to be used is to apply for a declaration that the proposed operation for sterilisation is lawful, and the following guidance was given as to the form to be followed in such proceedings:
   i. applications for a declaration that a proposed operation on or medical treatment for a patient can lawfully be carried out despite the inability of such patient to consent thereto should be by way of originating summons issuing out of the Family Division of the High Court;
   ii. the applicant should normally be those responsible for the care of the patient or those intending to carry out the proposed operation or other treatment, if it is declared to be lawful;
   iii. the patient must always be a party and should normally be a respondent. In cases in which the patient is a respondent the

patient's *guardian ad litem* should normally be the official solicitor. In any cases in which the official solicitor is not either the next friend or the guardian *ad litem* of the patient or an applicant he or she shall be a respondent;

iv. with a view to protecting the patient's privacy, but subject always to the judge's discretion, the hearing will be in chambers, but the decision and the reasons for that decision will be given in open court.

Mental disorder means mental illness, arrested or incomplete development of mind, psychopathic disorder and any other disorder or disability of mind and 'mentally disordered' shall be construed accordingly.

THE SIDAWAY CASE

The question of how much information and warning of risk which should be given to a patient was considered by the House of Lords in the case of *Sidaway v Gov of Bethlem Royal Hospital* [1985] AC 871. Lord Bridge indicated that a decision on what degree of disclosure of risks is best calculated to assist a particular patient to make a rational choice as to whether or not to undergo a particular treatment must primarily be a matter of clinical judgment. He was of the further opinion that a judge might in certain circumstances come to the conclusion that the disclosure of a particular risk was so obviously necessary to an informed choice that no reasonably prudent medical man would fail to make it. The kind of case which Lord Bridge had in mind would be an operation involving a substantial risk of grave adverse consequences. Lord Templeman stated that there was no doubt that a doctor ought to draw the attention of a patient to a danger which may be special in kind or magnitude or special to the patient. He further stated that it was the obligation of the doctor to have regard to the best interests of the patient but at the same time to make available to the patient sufficient information to enable the patient to reach a balanced judgment if he or she chooses to do so.

INDEX

Adoption
  residence order, no consent by
      person having   17
Affidavit
  format   103
  meaning   102
Area Child Protection Committee
  role of   86

Blood transfusion
  specific issue order, use of   25
Breast cancer
  treatment for   140

Care
  authorised person   119
  child in
      contact with   16, 21, 42
      definition   120
      parental responsibility for   9–13
  route into   39
Care and control order
  residence order, replacement
      by   16
Care contact order
  application for   42

statutory provision   16, 21
Care order
  application for, persons
      entitled   39
  definition   120
  duration of   44
  effect of   41
  grounds for   39–40
  interim   30, 43
  parental responsibility, applicant
      acquiring   10–12
  significant harm
      concept of   40
      definition   41
Child
  definitions   120–1
  medical treatment, consent to, *see*
      Medical treatment
  racial and religious needs   96
  residence order, application
      for   18–19
  rights of
      changing   7–8
      positive   7
  wishes and feelings, taking into
      account   2
Child abuse, *see also* Sexual abuse
  duty to prevent   57–8
  emotional   94
  initial suspicions of   87–8

Child abuse – *cont'd*.
  institutional   95
  investigation, inter-agency
    co-operation
    Area Child Protection Committee,
      role of   86
    child protection
      conferences   89–91
    need for   97
    parents, working with   88–9
    responsibilities   86
    sexual abuse, as to   92–4
    statutory provisions   85
    training in   86–7
    Working Together   86
  investigative examinations   83
  local authority's duty to
    prevent   57–8
  medical practitioner
    specialism, areas of   91
    suspicions of   87–8
  minority ethnic families   97
  neglect   57–8, 94–5
  non-sexual forms of   94–5
  other races and cultures, views
    of   96
  positive aspects of families,
    concentration on   89
  prevention, aim of   89–90
  protection from   85
  statutory intervention   97
  stress factors   96
Child assessment order
  application for
    person making   46
    steps towards   47–8
    when made   46–7
  assessment
    making   49
    multi-disciplinary   49
    overnight stays   50
    practitioner, presence of   49
    refusal to allow   51

  timing   50–51
  court, directions of   49–50
  emergency protection order, making
    of, on application   33
  guardian ad litem, role of   49
  local authority, duty of   45
  practice, pattern of   51–2
  process, recording   48
  race and culture   51
  sequence of action   46
  significant harm, where
    suspected   45–6
  use of   46
Child in need
  definition   120
  family
    definition   53
    role of   53, 55–6
  local authority
    accommodation by   56
    co-operation with   60
    family centres, provision of   57
    powers and duties of   54
    services, *see below* services for
    upbringing by family, promotion
      of   55–6
  medical practitioner, role
    of   59–60
  need, definitions of   53–4
  race and culture   58–9
  services for
    information about   55
    provision of   53
    range of   56
    voluntary agencies, of   60
Child protection
  family, understanding of   96
  gender, factor of   96
  legal procedures   6
  local measures   47
  sequence of action   46
Child protection conference
  management of   90

parents, involvement of, in 90
purpose of 89
recommended course of action,
    agreeing on 89
resolutions 91
Communication with children and
    adolescents
age-appropriate language 79–80
approach to 84
assumptions 79
child-centred approach 80–1
difficulties with 81–2
Gillick judgment, implications
    of 83
guardian ad litem, by 82
language problems 82
meaning 79
medical practitioner, by 82
play, through 81
sexual abuse, in case of 83
Contact
child in care, with 16, 21, 42
child in police protection,
    with 36–7
regulation of 19–20
scope of 19–20
preventing, use of prohibited steps
    order 19
Contact order
application for, leave for 18
contact, meaning 19
definition 19, 122
duration of 20
local authority, not used by 15–16
persons applying for 20
scope of 19–20
termination of 20
variation of 20
welfare of child, paramountcy
    of 15
Contraception
child under 16, advice to, without
    parental consent, on 8, ch 10

confidentiality, right to 83
County court
affidavits for 102–3
Custody order
residence order, replacement
    by 16

Data protection 131
Day care
local authority, provided by 57
race and culture 58–9
Disabilities, children with, *see also*
    Children in need
disability, definition 53–4, 122
local authority, powers and duties
    of 54
needs, assessing 60
register of 54–5
services for
information about 55
provision of 53
range of 55–6

Education supervision order 43, 123
Emergency protection order
accident and emergency department,
    examination of child in 32
child assessment order, made on
    application for 32
consequences of 31
definition 123
evidence in proceedings 31–2
execution of 31
medical practitioners, role
    of 31–3
parental responsibility, person
    having, acquiring 11–12
persons applying for 29
place of safety orders, superseding 29

Emergency protection order – *cont'd.*
  principles of Act, application
      of   33
  psychiatrists, role of   31–3
  significant harm to child, proof
      of   30
  temporary parental responsibility,
      acquisition of   31
  timing   30
  use of   33
Evidence
  affidavits   102–3
  court reports, *see* Medical reports
  exhibits   102, 106–7
  expert
    giving   116
    payment for   117
    preparation   113–14
    reports   113
    stages in   116
    witness, *see* Expert witness
  medical reports, *see* Medical reports
Expert witness
  court
    arrival at   114
    speaking outside   117
  evidence, giving   116
  magistrates and judges,
      addressing   115
  oath or affirmation   115
  organisations   118
  payment   117
  preparation   113–14
  tactics   115
  written report   113

Family assistance order
  definition   123
Family centre
  local authority, provision by   57
Family proceedings

court, definition   124
definition   123

Gillick
  competent   ch 10
  issues of parental consent   8, ch 10
Glossary   119–29
Guardian
  child subject to residence order,
      for   17
  parental responsibility, acquisition
      of   10–11
Guardian ad litem
  child assessment, role in   49–50
  communication with child   82
  court, advising   3
  medical examinations
    ascertaining wishes of child
        to   74, 82
    over-intrusive, guarding
        against   32
  records, etc, access to   3

Health education
  child care, role in   95
Health professionals
  child assessment, liaison
      during   47–8
  co-operation between   85
  emergency protection order,
      application for   29
  NHS guidance for   26
  medical information, confidentiality
      and disclosure of   131–4
  racial or cultural group, advice
      concerning   51
  relationships, breakdown in   48
Health records
  access to   131–4

High Court
  affidavits for   102–3
  powers of   24
Hospital
  emergency protection order, child
     subject to, being accommodated
     in   31–2

Local authority
  abuse and neglect, duty to
     prevent   57–8
  accommodation
    race and culture, taking into
      account   58–9
    responsibility to offer   56
    supportive mechanism, as   56
    voluntary basis, on   21
    written agreements   56
  care order, powers during   41
  child in need, services for, *see* Child
    in need
  contact order, not using   15–16
  day care, provision of   57
  definition   125
  children with disabilities, services
    for, *see* Disabilities, children
    with
  emergency protection order,
    application for   29
  family centres, provision of   57
  parental responsibility,
    acquiring   9, 11
  prohibited steps order,
    obtaining   23–4
  residence order, not using   15–16
  specific issue order, obtaining   23–4

Magistrates' court
  directions hearing in   2

family proceedings court   114
  preliminary hearing in   2
Medical examination and assessment
  arrangements for, court informed
    of   42
  care proceedings, order in   42–3
  child assessment order, in relation
    to   46
    making   49
    multi-disciplinary   49
    overnight stays   50
    practitioner, presence of   49
    race and culture   51
    refusal to allow   51
    timing   50–1
  child, informed refusal by
    care proceedings, in   42–3
    court overriding   75–6
    emergency protection order, in
      relation to   32
    rights as to   74–5
  Children Act provisions relating
    to   73–6
  consent, rules relating to   32, *see
    also* Medical treatment
  directions for   42–3
  emergency protection order,
    and   31–2
  expert evidence, for   99
  interim care or supervision order,
    on   43
  over-intrusive   32
  person carrying out   2
  practitioner, consent of   43
  repeated, order forbidding   43
  results of   2
  supervision order, directions
    with   42
  timetable for   2, 33
  venue for   2
Medical practitioner
  case conference, attending   33,
    48

Medical practitioner – *cont'd.*
  child abuse
    families, assessing   95
    investigation of   91
    referrals   94
    suspicions of   83, 88
  child assessment, presence
    during   49–50
  children in need, role in relation
    to   59–60
  communication with child   82–3
  emergency protection order
    accident and emergency
      department, examination of
      child in   32
    evidence in proceedings   31–2
    involvement in   33
    reports, supplying   33
    social worker, accompanying, to
      execute order   32
    timetable, preparation of   33
  enhancement of parental skills,
    encouragement of   88
  examination and assessment,
    agreement to   43
  medical treatment, agreement by, to
    carry out   43
  needs of child, assessing   59–61
  register of disabled children, advice
    on   55
  sexual abuse
    investigation of   91, 94
    referrals   94
    suspicions of   83, 88
  specialism   91
  treatment, unwilling to continue   43
Medical records
  format of   12
  guardian ad litem, access by   3
  person having parental
    responsibility, noting   70
Medical reports
  court, for

    acceptance of   99
    audio and video-tape recordings,
      use of   108
    checklist   104–5, 110–12
    Children Act reports and
      statements   101–2
    chronology/diary events   105
    confidentiality   110
    content   104–12
    events and dates   104
    exhibits   106–8
    format   101–3
    headings   104
    illustrations and photographs
      in   106
    jargon, avoiding   109
    notes and records   99–100
    observations and conclusions,
      information leading to   105–6
    personal information in   104
    preparation   101
    previous reports, bearing in
      mind   110
    questioning, account of   105–6
    references in   109
    summaries   109
    terminology   109
  emergency protection order, in
    relation to   33
Medical treatment
  blood transfusions   25
  breast cancer, consent for, of   140
  children and young people, consent
    for, of   137–8
  consent to
    adult, of   63–4
    anorexia, patient suffering
      from   65
    capacity to give, age for   64–5
    child under 16, of   66–9
    child 16 or over, of   64
    child, of   8, ch 10
    emergencies, in   63

emergency, whether situation
   is   76
full capacity   67
Gillick competence   66–9
guidance on   63–4
High Court inherent jurisdiction,
   use of   66
maternity services, for   140
mentally ill or disordered
   children, of   64, 69, 141–4
nearest relative, of   69
NHS guidance   26, 69
obtaining   136–7
parental responsibility, and   70
statutory provisions   139
sufficient understanding for   68
emergency protection order, role in
   course of   31–3
emergency situations, in   25–6
Gillick competent child,
   overriding   73
High Court, powers of   73
in-patient, regulation of   64
parents consenting but child
   refusing   72
parents refusing but child
   consenting to   71
patient, advising   135
practitioner carrying out   43
refusal of   138
right to refuse   65
risk, warning of   144
specific issue order, use of
   25–6
wishes of adult, courts
   respecting   66
without consent   139

Neglect
   child abuse, as   94–5
   duty to prevent   57–8

NSPCC
   care order, application for   39
   child assessment order, application
      for   45

Organ donation
   consent for   136

Parent
   child protection conference,
      involvement in   90
   definition   126
   legal status of   7
   parental responsibility, *see* Parental
      responsibility
Parental responsibility
   acquisition of
      emergency protection order, on
         grant of   11–12
      guardian, by   11
      local authority, by   9, 11
      natural father, by   10–11
      residence order, on
         obtaining   11, 17
   adoption, changing on   9
   agreement
      definition   126
      ending   11
      form of   11, 13
      use of   11
   birth of child, on   9
   care order, effect of   41
   definition   7, 126
   dispute over   11
   effect of   12
   emergency protection order, during
      duration of   31
   exercise of   17
   married parents, of   9–10

Parental responsibility – *cont'd.*
  medical records, indicated on   12,
    70
  medical treatment, consent to   70
  more than one person having   8
  non-parent with, definition   125
  order   11
  parent with   126
  persons other than parents
    having   9
  statutory obligations, effect on
    12
  transfer or surrender, incapable
    of   8
  unmarried father, of   10
  unmarried mother, of   10
Patients
  medical treatment, *see* Medical
    treatment
  teaching on   139
Place of safety order
  emergency protection order
    replacing   29
Police protection
  contact with child in   36–7
  extent of powers   35
  further action after implementation
    of   36
  inquiry into case   36
  persons to be informed of   36
  release from   36
  time-limits   35
  use of   35
Prohibited steps order
  contact, to prevent   19
  definition   26, 127
  duration of   27
  local authority, available to   23–4
  persons applying for   27
  scope of   27
  specific issue order, complementary
    to   23
  use of   23

Psychiatric examination and
    assessment
  arrangements for, court informed
    of   42
  attendance at   2
  care order, direction with
    42–3
  child assessment order, in relation
    to   46
  making   49
  multi-disciplinary   49
  overnight stays   50
  practitioner, presence of   49
  race and culture   51
  refusal to allow   51
  timing   50–1
  child, informed refusal by
    care proceedings, in   42–3
    court overriding wishes of
      75–6
    emergency protection order, in
      relation to   32
    rights as to   74–5
  Children Act provisions relating
    to   73–6
  consent to   32
  expert evidence, for   99
  interim care or supervision order,
    on   43
  person carrying out   2
  practitioner, agree to carry out   43
  repeated, order forbidding   43
  results of   2
  supervision order, directions
    with   42
  timetable for   2
  venue for   2
Psychiatric records
  guardian ad litem, access by
    3
Psychiatrist
  emergency protection order, role in
    course of   31–3

Race and culture
  accommodation by local authority,
      factors in   58–9
  child abuse, attitudes to   96–7
  child assessment, factors in   51
Residence order
  adoption, person having, not able to
      consent to   17
  application for
      child, by   19
      leave for   18–19
      persons entitled as of right   18
  child in care, in respect of   16
  child subject to, taken out of
      jurisdiction   18
  definition   16, 127
  duration of   19
  local authority, not used
      by   15–16
  more than one person, in favour
      of   16
  parental responsibility, person
      having, acquiring   11, 17
  person not parent having, limitations
      of   17–18
      scope of   16–17
      surname of child, no power to
          change   18
  welfare of child, paramountcy
      of   15

Section 8 orders, *see also* Contact
      order; Prohibited steps order;
      Residence order; Specific issue
      order
  conjunction, made in   23
  creation of   15
  power of court to make   23
  use of   15
Sexual abuse, *see also* Child abuse
  investigation of

gender, race, culture and religion,
      taking into account   94
  medical intervention   92
  non-abusing parent or carer,
      involvement of   93
  other children, abuse by   93
  police and social worker,
      interview by   92
  investigative examinations   83
  non-abusing parent, involvement
      of   93
  other children, by   93
  perpetrators
      men as   96
  removal from home   93
  psychosomatic symptoms   94
  urgent medical intervention   92
Social service
  files, access to   131–2
Specific issue order
  definition   24, 128
  dispute by persons with parental
      responsibility, application in
      case of   8–9
  duration of   26
  local authority, available to   23–4
  medical treatment, in relation
      to   25–6
  persons applying for   26
  problems arising, use of   25
  prohibited steps order,
      complementary to   23
  scope of   25
  use of   23
Statutory obligations
  child, in relation to   12
Sterilisation
  consent, issue of   64, 143–4
Supervision order
  authorised person   119
  definition   128
  duration of   44
  education   43

Supervision order – *cont'd*.
  effect of   42
  grounds for   40
  interim   43
  significant harm
    concept of   40
    definition   41
Surname
  child's, change of   18

Tape recordings
  evidence, as   108
Tissue donation
  consent for   141

Underlying principles
  delay, avoidance of   1–2
  non-intervention, principle of   4
  partnership and co-operation,
    concepts of   1
  person, child as   2

welfare of child, paramountcy
    of   1–3, 15

Video recordings
  evidence, as   108
Voluntary agencies
  children in need, services for   60
  family centres, provision of   57

Wardship
  current use of, in medical
      treatment   ch 10
  curtailment of   24, ch 10
Welfare
  checklist   3
  family proceedings, questions
      arising in   15
  paramount consideration, as   1–3,
      15
  positive duty to safeguard, not
      implied   8